Over the last few years, I've sought out the wisdom of Meredyth Fletcher again and again. Her ability to tie the physical elements of health with the spiritual never ceases to amaze me. Her book is a grace-filled manual that makes health—and getting back to the beauty of health—approachable yet sustainable. I love the blend of practicality and inspiration and Meredyth's ability to lean away from the trends to press deeper into the eternal impact of cultivating a healthy lifestyle. Be sure to keep a pen and notebook nearby—you'll take lots of notes as you go!

HANNAH BRENCHER, author of *Fighting Forward* and *Come Matter Here*

Finding a well-integrated approach to health—especially one written from a biblical perspective—is so difficult, but Meredyth has given us just that! In a clear and balanced way, she takes what can be a very complex and "science-y" topic and brings the main principles to light. Her personal experience combined with her education bring a powerful combo to each page! I came away with a renewed focus on and energy toward health and healing from the inside out.

CLARE SMITH, leadership and life coach

Meredyth gracefully illustrates how God's design for our bodies is perfect and full of abundance. She details how we can enjoy the process of nourishing our bodies, take delight in the foods we eat, and honor God at the same time. *The (Good) Food Solution* will help you feel great so that you can walk into the plans God has for you daily!

CAROLINE POTTER, functional nutritional therapy practitioner and creator of Flourish: Cultivating Conscious Living

In an age of quick fixes, fad diets, and conflicting nutritional advice, most women (like me) are left confused and disillusioned! Into this noise steps Meredyth Fletcher with her timely and much-needed guidance that is wise and full of grace. *The (Good) Food Solution* offers readers clear answers . . . as well as peace, wholeness, and a loving respect for the bodies God gave us. I'm thankful for Meredyth's wisdom; this is the book I've been searching for!

MARIAN JORDAN ELLIS, host of *This Redeemed Life* podcast and author of *Garden to Garden*

Take everything you learned as a kid about nutrition and throw it out the window! Reading Meredyth's book helped give me a clean slate and a fresh start on all things nutrition. Meredyth stepped on my toes in the best way while being full of grace and love. As a busy mom of three kids, I appreciate how this book helped shift my thinking about food and the important ways it fuels our bodies, not only physically but also emotionally, mentally, and spiritually. I'm excited to get back to the basics and start implementing practical ways to get around the table with my family. I also really enjoyed the practical tips and "Digging Deeper" questions at the end of each chapter, which would lead to a great book discussion for any small group.

JENN HAMM, event coordinator at Living Proof Ministries

Meredyth's approach to holistic health is paving a path of freedom for so many. Not only is she guiding us through a mindful and meaningful way to redeem and refine our health, she's also pointing us to the gospel, which is everything because it's what rectifies our souls. She needs to proclaim this message of hope and healing from the mountaintops, and this book being out in the world is just the beginning of the echoes of freedom that will be heard and felt for generations.

ELIZABETH COX, founder of Refined Business Collective,
Karpós client, and business coach specializing in holistic refinement

Few people can bring together the academics of nutrition, the wisdom of sound theological teaching, and the heart of counseling around the subject of food like Meredyth can. In *The (Good) Food Solution*, this combination is as life-giving as you would imagine because Meredyth is the rare type of author you don't just trust but enjoy!

LANIE BETH SINCLAIR, master of biblical and theological studies

When I picked up *The (Good) Food Solution*, I was not expecting to be touched so deeply by a message on health and nutrition. There is so much goodness in this book! Meredyth Fletcher's approach is holistic, it's genuine, and it's rooted in biblical wisdom. I am grateful for this inspiring and helpful guide that makes taking the next step in pursuing a healthy lifestyle so inviting and attainable.

LEIGH KOHLER, cofounder and president of the
Freedom Church Alliance

Meredyth is the gracious and educated guide we need for this journey. If you feel blissfully ignorant or overwhelmed about food, this book will give you the confidence to make lifelong positive changes for God's glory instead of your own.

VALERIE WOERNER, author of *Pray Confidently and Consistently*
and creator of Val Marie Paper prompted prayer journal

The (Good) Food Solution

MEREDYTH FLETCHER LPC-A NTP

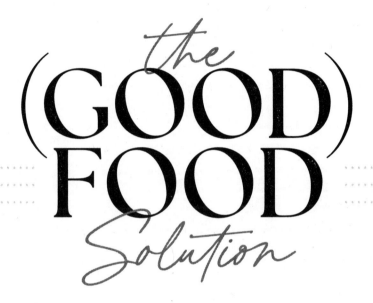

the (GOOD) FOOD Solution

A SHAME-FREE

NUTRITIONAL JOURNEY

TO FOOD FREEDOM,

SPIRITUAL NOURISHMENT

& WHOLE-BODY HEALTH

TYNDALE
REFRESH®

Think Well. Live Well. Be Well.

Visit Tyndale online at tyndale.com.

Visit Meredyth Fletcher at karposwellness.com.

30	29	28	27	26	25	24
7	6	5	4	3	2	1

To my husband, Daniel, and our babies.

My personal journey toward health and wholeness began when I was single because I knew that one day you would be the most special part of my life, and I wanted to show up as my whole self. Little did I know that, because of you, I would come to know Jesus and the fullness of healing and life better—beyond measure.

Daniel,

you are the most incredibly inspiring human I've ever known. Your desire and drive to live a healthy life—mind, body, and soul—are unmatched, and I'm grateful that you lead our family in a way that promotes freedom and healing. I'm also grateful for your insane ability to cook deliciously nourishing foods in the kitchen.

My babies,

you are a dream come true and absolute miracles to me. I promise to commit to a life of health and healing, no matter what it takes, in order to mother and nurture you to the best of my human ability. You're worth every bit of what it takes, and I love you more than words can say.

Medical Disclaimer

The health and nutritional information in this book is intended for educational purposes only. The author's information and opinions are based on years of research and clinical education, but they should not be used as a substitute for professional medical advice, diagnosis, and treatment. Readers are advised to consult their own physicians and practitioners for specific individual help concerning any health issue and to talk with them before beginning a new eating program.

Contents

Introduction

"Why do I feel so sluggish?"

"Why am I always anxious?"

"Why can't I lose weight?"

"Why can't I sleep through the night?"

These are just some of the questions I hear from new clients. Often they come to me with one primary health concern that they've tried to solve on their own for months or years. They may have thought they'd landed on the solution when they looked around and saw someone who had seemingly gained new energy, overcome depression, or lost weight. They diligently adopted the same strategy and started off with great expectations. Sometimes the new diet or exercise program worked for a while, but inevitably it stalled out. Then hope was renewed with the discovery of yet another eating plan or workout. The cycle began again.

Perhaps you can relate. You're either desperate to find answers or so tired of the struggle that you are tempted to give up altogether. Whatever the battle looks like for you—whether over the food on your plate, your fear of or obsession about eating, or your despair at not seeing results—you can discover the freedom you're looking for.

Though I'm now a nutritional therapy practitioner and counselor, I was once caught in the same never-ending cycle of trying the latest diet while also trying to figure out my body. I used to think God must be disappointed in me for focusing on my physical wellness and trying to lose weight. I assumed that He wanted me to focus on more "holy" pursuits and give any leftover attention to my body. I assumed that physical wellness should never be top of mind but more of an afterthought. Wrong.

Though my original motives may have been confused, I now know that God created all of me—body, mind, and spirit—to flourish. Once I realized that God not only cares about my health but that He created real foods to perfectly meet my body's needs, I made it my mission to learn all I could about nutrition and then teach others how to fuel their beautiful bodies in the way He designed.

God wired us as humans with the *need* to tend to our physical bodies each day. If we don't care for the physical bodies He gave us, how will we have the strength and energy to show up fully on this earth? If we lack the proper fuel and discipline needed to maintain a healthy life, how are we supposed to obey His commands to love Him and love others? That doesn't mean we have to live up to impossible standards; life can be difficult, and some days I still struggle to figure out what works best. But I've discovered that when I fuel my body with whole foods, I feel great and am able to show up well for myself and others.

The news gets even better. Not only did God design us to survive, but He wants us to thrive. Jesus promised His followers: "I came that they may have and enjoy life, and have it in abundance [to the full, till it overflows]" (John 10:10, AMP). God created food that's designed to fill our bodies with the nutrients they need; He gives us His truth to fill our minds as we take other thoughts captive (2 Corinthians 10:5); and He provides His Spirit to fill our entire beings. This is the way to the abundant life that God offers.

Regardless of the health goal you're after, this is what it comes down to: allowing your body, mind, and spirit the time and space they need to heal. Nothing will work unless they are tended to at the foundation. No amount of sun and water can remedy a plant with dying roots; likewise, no diet based on calorie burning or restriction will bring healing to your entire being.

In *The (Good) Food Solution*, we'll consider what foods will best serve every part of you, along with other healthy practices that will promote healing in your body, mind, and spirit. Because the path to health and healing starts in your gut, we will also look at the incredible and intricate way God designed it to serve as the gateway to the nutrients your body needs. Finally, we will explore just how much God longs for you to be whole and what it looks like to invite Him into this journey.

At the end of each chapter, you'll find tips and questions so that you can begin applying the concepts in this book. The Whole-Body Health Protocol, which is designed to help you put into practice what you've learned, is included as an appendix. I've also provided recipes to show you how to incorporate whole and healthy foods into your snacks and meals.

My goal is to ensure that you feel more empowered to nourish your body and be kind to yourself. I want to encourage you to invite God to be a deeper part of your healing and to fully show up for your own life. Get ready to dig up anything that is rotting and replant yourself near streams of living water where you can flourish for good (Psalm 1:3)!

1

FOOD FOR THOUGHT

HOW DID WE GET HERE WITH NUTRITION?

The strains of Southern bluegrass filled my tiny SUV as I drove along I-40 toward Houston. A recent college graduate, I was leaving my hometown in Kentucky for a chance to start a new chapter of life. When noon rolled around several hours into my drive, I ripped open a bag of Cheetos, washing them down with Diet Mountain Dew. To me, this was the ideal lunch—cheap comfort food that, in limited quantities, would keep me thin. That was important: I wanted my jeans to be a certain size, and I needed to keep control over my very out-of-control life.

Though I'd navigated a rocky couple of years, I hadn't always been that concerned about my diet. In fact, growing up I barely gave any thought to what or how much I ate. I didn't have to. I spent hours in the gym or on the ball field, throwing myself into whatever sport was in season. As a result, I could eat pretty much whatever I wanted.

Then one day in college, my roommate picked up a pair of my jeans and exclaimed, "Is *this* really your jean size?!" I was genuinely stumped. I had never thought about my jean size until right then—the moment that changed everything. Suddenly burgers, pizza, macaroni and cheese, and enormous salads were off-limits. From then on I stuck to drinking coffee and eating whole wheat crackers and apples almost exclusively. I prided myself on seeing how long I could go before I felt hungry in the morning. Coffee kept me feeling full for hours. When the hunger pangs kicked in, I would eat an apple. A normal dinner consisted of exactly fourteen wheat crackers and maybe some grilled chicken. I would head straight to the gym after eating to shave those calories off if I hadn't already "stored up" negative calories from the thirty to sixty minutes I spent on a cardio machine every morning. That year, I dropped four pant sizes and about thirty pounds. I became completely obsessed . . . and miserable. I shed the unwanted pounds but at the cost of an unsustainable lifestyle that left me exhausted, overwhelmed, and completely out of touch with my body.

Without knowing it, I was treating my body just about as badly as when I ate whatever I wanted. Proper nourishment wasn't my focus; in fact, that never even crossed my mind. Instead, I watched to see what the people I wanted to look like were doing and assumed that's what I should do too. I was ignoring and mistreating the internal system God had created to nourish and nurture every part of me.

If you can relate to any part of my story, you're in the right place, and I'm glad you're here. Rather than focusing on your outward appearance, do you long to see your body and nutritious foods as good gifts from God and to know that He loves you just as you are? I know that your quest for a better body might have started out innocently. You thought it would be nice—harmless or even healthy—to lose a few (or many) pounds to feel better in your own skin. There's nothing wrong with that. You looked around to see what someone else was doing to reach or keep their goal weight. Whether it was a coworker eating the same lunch of tuna and carrot sticks or the friend extolling her premade protein shakes, you thought you'd found your solution. It would work or it wouldn't, but even if it did, the results never lasted. What gives?

I understand how frustrating it can be to feel like you're eating all the right foods and getting nowhere. Although you may decide to seek help from a practitioner or experiment with short-term elimination diets to pinpoint the culprits, in many cases, small and/or chronic ailments can be reduced or even eliminated by (1) focusing on eating real foods and (2) working to improve the health of your gut environment.

Throughout this book, we will take a look at how to end the mental, physical, and emotional cycle of the dreaded food battle for good. Food should be desired and pleasurable. Food should work for you and not against you. And if you feel like it hasn't been up to this point, don't lose hope. The good news is this: God created a world full of nourishing food that is designed to provide health and wholeness. Before we get into the basics of food and gut health, then, let's consider what we were created to eat—and how we moved so far away from eating as God intended.

TEMPTED BY FOOD FROM THE BEGINNING

When we choose to host people in our homes, we want to offer our best, giving our guests special attention and hospitality. That requires forethought and preparation. Before the Lord even created human beings, He, too, took time to prepare a hospitable place for us. Only after creating the light, water, sun, moon, stars, plants, and animals—laying a beautiful foundation for the right kind of nourishment—did God create man. God thought of food as fuel before He made man to need it. Adam was made from the dust of the ground—the very place where God had created plants to grow for people's nourishment. After making man, God planted a garden and instructed Adam to tend it (Genesis 2:5-15). The Lord gave Adam free rein of his home—except for a single tree. God invited Adam to enjoy everything else in the Garden but warned him that if he ate from the tree of the knowledge of good and evil, he would die.

Realizing that it wasn't good for Adam to be alone, God made him a helper, Eve. The Garden of Eden gave them full access to abundant life. There they could dwell with God and feast on everything that the earth provided.

Together Adam and Eve, the first man and woman, were to work and sustain the land. Since we are made from the same stuff, it makes sense that we, too, need good food from plants (and animals) in order to function well and heal. Notice that growing and preparing nourishing food has taken time, effort, and work from the very beginning.

Before the fall of man, feasting was beautiful, life-giving, and sustaining. Then Satan in the guise of a serpent entered the Garden and convinced Eve that God was trying to keep something from her and Adam by making one tree off-limits. That tree's fruit looked good, and Eve wanted to be wise like God, so she ate and gave some to Adam. Their disobedience had cosmic implications, but from their story, we also see that the narrative of self-control and discipline around food is not new. As Joel Soza, an author and professor of biblical studies, notes, "Food, the very substance that gave our first ancestors life in God's garden, became the very object that led to their death."[1]

Adam and Eve's disobedience led to immediate consequences. God told the man and woman:

> Cursed is the ground because of you;
>> through painful toil you will eat food from it
>> all the days of your life.
> It will produce thorns and thistles for you,
>> and you will eat the plants of the field.
> By the sweat of your brow
>> you will eat your food
> until you return to the ground,
>> since from it you were taken;
> for dust you are
>> and to dust you will return.
>
> GENESIS 3:17-19

If we were made from the ground and we return to the ground, then what do we do with the in-between? How do we live and breathe from ground to ground? We work. In today's society, not all of us can be farmers who live off the land, cultivating plants and raising animals, but we can get to know the farmers near us. We can get to know the soil around us.

HOW DID WE GET HERE?

Of course, after the Fall, the nutrients that originally could be harvested with minimal effort now required hard labor. As we'll see, people have always looked for ways to make food production easier, and today's modern, quick-food lifestyle has taken us far away from how it was supposed to be. Not only do we forget the command to work for our food, but many nutrients are getting lost in prepackaged food-like substances that aren't "real." Our bodies lack many of the necessary enzymes to break down these foods. It makes sense that people are getting so sick.

While we still expect to enjoy and be satisfied by our food, we often fail to honor God's command to eat real food. Instead, we've spent *years* trying to figure out how to cut corners for faster food, more money, and prettier bodies. If we go back to the beginning, we see that in order for food to fuel our bodies the way God intended, we have a responsibility to uphold—one that requires thoughtfulness, time management, discipline, and deep gratitude. A responsibility to think theologically about food.

Let's begin by considering what happened. How did we get here? Did our ancestors have this much trouble with food? I would be willing to bet that they labored but not like us. Their struggles involved tilling the soil and growing grain, as well as hunting animals and catching fish. They combined hard physical labor with a diet taken largely from the ground. In other words, they treated their bodies as God created them to do. They sometimes had to migrate from hot to cold climates, depending on where food was growing in any given season. Their crops were more susceptible to damage from droughts, insect invasions, and early frost.

Today, processed foods are cheap and readily available, and though we still work hard and at breakneck speed, we don't use our bodies as much. Our concerns are more likely linked to seeking convenience and wondering how to find tasty food, fast. At the same time, we're flooded with information on everything from weight loss to muscle toning, hormone balancing, thyroid support—you name it. In the midst of all these changes, our society is genuinely confused and ignorant about what real food is. That has led to doubt and confusion around what we want, need, and desire for our bodies. We end up living with shame over our bodies because we are relying on fake substitutes that pretend to be nutritious but deny us the real nutrients our bodies need.

Of course, the dramatic differences between the diet of the Israelites and people today didn't happen overnight; in fact, let's look at five turning points that affected the way we eat.

Five milestones that influenced food production

AGRICULTURAL REVOLUTION (14,000-2,000 YEARS AGO)

Our earliest ancestors were hunters and gatherers, but the agricultural revolution took place as people learned to domesticate plants and animals. Populations began to grow, and rather than wandering in search of food, people established permanent settlements. These agricultural and technological advances were in the baby stages of development but enabled greater production and efficiency when preparing food.[2]

INTRODUCTION OF REFINED SUGAR (APPROXIMATELY 1600s)

Although sugar had been processed in India and the Middle East for centuries, European producers expanded the industry, developing technologies, such as waterwheels, that enabled them to crush sugarcane and then boil down real cane sugar to produce a sweet, crystalized substance. Vitamins and minerals were lost in the process. Unfortunately, the European and American slave trade supported the labor-intensive production process. Several hundred years ago, refined sugar was rare and expensive, so it didn't cause a huge nutritional problem, but advances in sugar production have led to greater problems today.[3]

INDUSTRIAL REVOLUTION (EARLY 1800s-MID 1900s)

Once large factories came on the scene, the centralized mass production of foods became possible. To increase the shelf life of food items, manufacturers developed processes that stripped many nutrients from the foods. This revolution was largely driven by a desire to increase productivity and economic gains.

WORLD WAR II (1940s)

Because of the need to feed US allies and troops on the front lines, the war created an even more pressing desire for food preservation. While this led to a decrease in the nutrient value of many foods, experts in nutrition did begin counseling citizens on how to avoid food waste and preserve vitamins and minerals when cooking fruits and vegetables.[4]

CONVENIENCE AND FAST FOODS (POSTWAR PERIOD TO PRESENT)

Manufacturers used their new knowledge of preservation to capitalize on convenience and economics. Advances in technology, including assembly-line production and a national interstate highway system, encouraged the development of food manufacturers and fast-food franchises that prioritized speed and taste over nutrition.[5] The development of chemical flavorings and advances in processing and preserving technologies—along with a demand for ready-to-eat meals due to busy lifestyles—meant an expansion in convenience foods.[6] Essentially little to no nutrients are left in fast food and convenience items because of the way they've been processed.

I realize that I just gave you a crash course in the history of food production. So where does that leave us now? Food is certainly cheaper and easier to come by; however, here is just some of the fallout:

- produce and meats with impurities and contaminants like heavy metals, pesticides, parasites, and unwanted bacteria, which are introduced into food during the process of getting it from the farm to the table[7]
- meats with steroids and antibiotics
- milk filled with hormones
- man-made foods with toxins, artificial sweeteners, artificial additives, MSG, and preservatives

We were not made to rush through our days and mindlessly eat microwaved meals and frozen pizzas. Nor do we need to.

WHERE DO WE GO FROM HERE?

Before we look more closely at what I mean by "real foods," nutrients, and gut health, I propose three steps to approach food and fuel our bodies in the way God intended.

Be thankful

The further we get from tilling our own land, the easier it is to forget to receive each meal God provides with genuine thankfulness. Yet the abundance of nutrient-rich, readily available foods isn't anything we should take for granted. Gratitude is a huge part of how our bodies heal and grab hold of the redemptive promises God offers. (We dive deeper into the science behind this in later chapters.) It is one way we fulfill the greatest commandment:

> Jesus replied, "'You must love the LORD your God with all your heart, all your soul, and all your mind.' This is the first and greatest commandment. A second is equally

important: 'Love your neighbor as yourself.' The entire
law and all the demands of the prophets are based on
these two commandments."
MATTHEW 22:37-40, NLT

Slow down

God designed our bodies to optimally digest when we are calm and
relaxed, and they prioritize digestion when we are in this serene
state of being. The brain physically triggers the body's process of
breaking down food when we start to think about and smell food.
Upon awakening these senses, we begin to salivate at the thought
of an upcoming meal or snack. The brain immediately sends signals through the nervous system to the gut so that it is prepared
and ready to receive and digest food.

When we are in a stressed state, on the other hand, our bodies
prioritize survival, not digestion. If you've ever eaten while standing up, in front of a computer, or driving a car, you likely felt
bloated and icky afterward. That's because your body didn't have
the time and space it needed to prepare for proper digestion. We
will explore this further in chapter 9.

Eat locally produced foods

Eating locally is also another important factor in allowing our
bodies to heal. Eating an apple from your local orchard or farmer's
market will be different from eating precut apples from the grocery
store. Here's how: When you pick and eat an apple from an apple
tree that has had little to no chemical spraying, you are consuming the fruit in its purest form. This apple is rich in nutrients and
perfect for consumption—allowing you to receive all the benefits
from those nutrients. It's been grown properly and sustained naturally just the way God intended.

When you buy precut apple slices portioned in individual bags from the grocery store, you're not receiving all the nutritional benefits the original apple had.[8] Let's say you live in Colorado, but the apple was grown in Washington. Someone else picked that apple before it was thrown on a truck and transported to the store. You have no idea what it's been sprayed with and no control over its care. You don't know how well its temperature was controlled as it made its way to the processing plant, where it was perfectly cut, soaked in something to prevent browning, and individually bagged. With all the changes this apple has undergone, its nutrients have been stripped away little by little. This means its nutritional value has gone down, and you won't reap all the benefits the apple once had to offer.

Thanking God, slowing down, and eating what is cultivated from the ground, as close to you as possible, are great ways to nourish your body. Such holy nourishment takes time and careful tending, but it will genuinely feed your mind, body, and soul.

Let's talk about how we ended up here. *Why* is eating the right food so hard? What if I told you it's not actually that complicated?

GET REAL!

As basic as it sounds, learning to distinguish real food from what I call "fake food" is critical to better health. After all, food manufacturers often slap labels on their products that are intended to convince you that their products are nutritional. But what are the characteristics of real food—aside from the fact that they usually bear no label at all? Look for foods that are

- whole and unprocessed
- free of synthetic chemicals

- local, fresh, and varied with the seasons
- as wild and sustainable as possible
- humanely processed
- lacking complicated labels or flashy brands
- good for a limited time due to short shelf life

True or false? Examples of real food include apples, carrots, and chicken. Answer? It all depends. According to my definition, an apple you pick from the tree or from the grocery produce aisle is real food, while slices packaged in plastic are not. Hormone- and antibiotic-free free-range chicken is real, but frozen breaded chicken nuggets are not.

Real food is God-given from the ground and the animals He created. Real foods *are* ingredients; they don't *have* ingredients. As a result, real food often requires preparation. In such foods, God gave us everything we need for optimal health and fully functioning bodies.

What about all the foods in the middle of the grocery store in packaged boxes, jars, and bags? Those "foods" are actually not real. Almost all these products contain processed ingredients, using things like flour, sugar, or corn. In addition, for something to become shelf stable, manufacturers add ingredients to preserve its freshness and contents. These preservatives, gums, and fillers are not sourced from real foods but are synthetic products that the body has an extremely hard time digesting.[9] These additives are what make foods "fake." They're food-like substances that your body doesn't fully recognize as fuel.

Consuming those foods on a regular basis wreaks havoc on your system, leading to poor digestive function. Digestive organs become burdened, detoxification pathways become compromised, and the body has a hard time absorbing and distributing nutrients appropriately, leading to a host of unwanted health issues. If the body is trying too hard to do something it was *not* created to do, it becomes too tired to do what it was *designed* to do. Our bodies need real food for real nourishment.

I'm not saying you can never again enjoy a sweet treat or indulge in a processed food that brings you joy. What I am saying is that consuming these foods day in and day out will make you sick. Your digestive system needs to be tended to and healed before you can truly enjoy those indulgent foods. You will find much wisdom by considering the way God designed food as part of His creation.

HOW DO WE START?

God gifted us with delicious foods from the earth to nourish us. How about learning today to deeply love food again? How about if we stop assuming that food is the enemy of our bodies and souls? What if we stop fearing food and start believing that nutritious foods are good gifts from God and that He loves our bodies? What if we could experience true happiness while feasting instead of leaving a meal and repeatedly saying how much we overindulged in these delicious foods with our loved ones or how much we just messed up? The truth is, we were made to need food—there's no way around it. Let's make peace with the food we were given in order to live to the fullest.

Somewhere along the way, we've lost the love and theology of real food, and it's time to get it back. It's time to put art, truth, and life back into real food while learning about nutrients and how they add value to our bodies and our lives. Food should be enjoyed. Food should be delicious. Food should be eaten with thankfulness, remembrance, and a holy reverence for the One who gifted us with it. Food should be believed in—that it will be kind to us and help us see alignment and results, as long as we have the tools for sifting through the lies and knowledge for how to feed the body well. Let's have confidence in food again and take the first step on the path toward a beautiful relationship with food and our bodies.

Tips for Eating Good Food in the Right Way

1. Give thanks before you eat. Acknowledging God's gift of wholesome, nutritious food before eating will make you more present to your meal, which means you will enjoy it more.
2. Sit down while eating. To digest food properly, your body needs to be in a calm state, which it won't be when you eat in a hurry or on the go.
3. Chew slowly. Your digestive system won't have to work as hard if your food is thoroughly chewed before you swallow.
4. Stay away from the center of the grocery store, except to pick up organic flavor enhancers, like herbs and spices or condiments made without sugar.
5. Try locally sourcing meat and produce from a nearby farm or farmer's market in order to best nourish your body and support farmers who are doing the laborious work of providing food for others.

digging deeper

1. Which of the following made you pick up this book? Check all that apply.

   ☐ Desire to control food cravings
   ☐ GI issues (such as bloating, acid reflux, gassiness)
   ☐ Dissatisfaction with weight
   ☐ Mood swings
   ☐ Other: _____

2. Do you enjoy food or stress over it? Why?
3. Do you prepare your own meals? Why or why not? If not, is that something you're willing to do in order to be in control of what is happening inside your body?
4. Before you eat, how can you make space to offer thanksgiving to God for the foods He has provided?
5. What is one thing you have learned about the power of real food and nutrients to help heal your body?

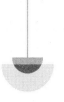

2

GUT CHECK

THE "INSIDE" STORY

When I left for Houston in my little SUV, I had no real plan. I had one acquaintance there and knew not another soul. After two full days of travel—nearly sixteen hours in the car—and a quick overnight in a hotel in Texarkana, I pulled up to my new home early in the evening. It took me all of fifteen minutes to unload my SUV and sit on my new bed. *What have I just done?* I closed my eyes and then looked around the room. *Did I really do this? Have I lost my mind?*

I had $120 and a few small gift cards to my name. I had come up short in my efforts to land a job before I got to Houston. My car payment wouldn't be due for another four weeks, so I figured if I could pay my cell phone bill and subsist on popcorn and peanut butter, I had some time to figure things out. I was ready for a head-down, knees-down kind of living. I was caught somewhere in the middle of intense anxiety and trusting God completely. I *wanted* to trust God, but also I *had* to trust God; there were no other options.

Nobody fully understood the life I had left behind in Kentucky. Growing up, I realized that some of the people who were supposed to love me most weren't able to do so. Though they tried with every ounce of their being, they just couldn't do it. Then, once I made the decision to leave, I was told I'd never make it on my own. That didn't stop me. I was a people pleaser and loved those around me, but I felt as if I was wilting under the unhealthy behaviors and patterns in my hometown. If I stayed there, I would not truly be able to heal.

I left Kentucky feeling I had no other option, even though I'd been told the job I really wanted in Texas wouldn't be available for a long time. Then, incredibly, my first morning in Houston, I received a call and was offered that very job. The position had unexpectedly opened the night before, so I could start the following Monday. I calculated quickly and realized that by the time I was trained and received my first paycheck, I would be able to pay my bills and make a full grocery run. That phone call felt like God catching me and lovingly whispering, "I told you."

Even so, my health issues continued. When I moved away from home, I didn't realize that, along with my suitcase, I was hauling my distorted thinking and bad habits to Texas. By skipping breakfast, drinking only coffee and water, and making apples and wheat crackers the staples of my diet, I had been slowly destroying my gut. The digestive system and the brain are so deeply connected that not only was I making it harder for my body to metabolize and use nutrients, but I was also making it more difficult for my body to process my emotional pain.

Not surprisingly, my troubles didn't disappear simply because I had moved. I still had trouble sleeping, and I often felt as if I was dragging through the day. I cycled through fad diet after fad diet with disappointing results.

Because I'd started looking at food as the enemy, I second-guessed everything I put in my mouth. I was left feeling hopeless and emotionally drained. But not long after I arrived in Houston, I realized I couldn't outrun those issues, so I began working with a therapist and a nutritionist. That's when I realized that the key to health and wholeness had been inside me the entire time. God created our bodies to optimize the nutrients they take in—and once we understand His design, we can begin to heal our bodies, minds, and spirits.

WHAT'S THE GUT GOT TO DO WITH IT?

It's frustrating to feel like you're eating all the right things without seeing the results you were hoping for. It doesn't have to be this way! If you feel like you're eating the best you possibly can without losing weight or feeling better, it's easy to assume that food is the cause. Although it can certainly contribute to digestive issues, food is most often *not* the root issue. Instead, many health conditions are signs that your digestive system is out of whack. In fact, how well it functions is quite possibly the most crucial factor of your health journey.

Though we tend to take it for granted, our gut, or gastrointestinal tract, is absolutely essential and central to ensuring that every system in our body works efficiently. In the next few chapters, we'll dive into food and nutrition, and later I'll introduce you to the Whole-Body Health Protocol, which can help restore well-being to your digestive system so you can healthfully and appropriately usher your body into the kind of abundant living you've always wanted.

But just as you can't drive a car until you learn the basics about how its various systems operate, it's difficult to understand how to get the most from your body until you understand how it works. So let me give you a quick flyover tour of the way your body takes in the energy, fuel, and nutrients it needs. Your digestive system breaks down and digests food, absorbs nutrients, eliminates waste and toxins, and sends signals to other parts of the body so they function properly.[1]

The gastrointestinal tract—with its impressive list of responsibilities—includes the mouth, throat, esophagus, stomach, small intestine, and large intestine. The liver, gallbladder, and pancreas are connected to the GI tract via small individual ducts, or tubes. The illustration below shows how they are connected.

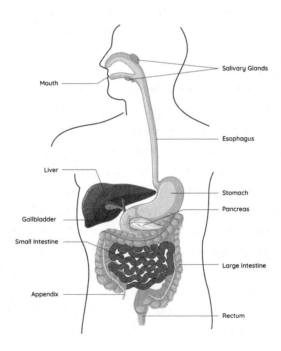

Another critical piece of your GI tract is the gut microbiome in the intestines. This is the pathway responsible for distributing nutrients across the intestinal barrier and into the bloodstream. When each individual organ and tissue performs its own delegated assignment together with the rest, the body can run optimally. Almost every symptom the body experiences, good and bad, begins in the gut.

Because the digestive system's two primary functions are to process and deliver nutrients to every part of your body and to identify and eliminate harmful toxins and bacteria from your gastrointestinal tract, you need to consider two questions when evaluating your health. First, it's important to ask, *Is my body absorbing nutrients?* Second, *Is my body eliminating toxins?*[2] These two simple questions can help you wade through the confusion and bring your body into alignment. In the coming chapters you will learn ways to identify whether or not your body is effectively doing both.

If the GI tract isn't working correctly, trendy diets and elimination plans will never work. Your gut is connected to everything, and the pathways from the gut microbiome to the bloodstream need to be clear in order for nutrients to be dispersed and opportunistic bacteria and toxins eliminated. Getting nutrients through a compromised gut is like trying to get a message to someone through a staticky phone line. The other person can hear you, but it's hard to really decipher what you're saying. Find good reception, and then they can hear you clear as day. Likewise, when your detoxification pathways are unobstructed, nutrients can be delivered where they're needed, and toxins and waste can be removed from your system.

Since the body is always detoxing, you just need to make sure the pathways are free of static. Even a healthy person's gut will have some opportunistic bacteria and toxins, but they should be flushed out of the body through sweating and going to the bathroom. If the pathways are not clear channels, you may experience issues like brain fog, hormone imbalances, skin issues, weight loss plateaus, inflammation, joint pain, autoimmune diseases, food sensitivities, parasites, digestive issues, insomnia, vomiting, infertility, and more. That's because the distribution of nutrients is stifled, opportunistic bacteria can grow, and the toxins you've been exposed to as a result of daily living can cycle around. At that point, it becomes an uphill battle to see results. You need to clear the pathways and support healing so that nutrients the body was designed to take in can have their desired effect.

THE ANSWER INSIDE YOU

What you eat and how well your body absorbs nutrients determine how efficiently the gut sends nutrients and signals elsewhere to the body. That is why, of all your bodily systems, the GI tract is arguably the most important to tend to. When things go awry, the healing priority becomes the gut. And when things are going well, it's important to tend to it in order to maintain whole-body health. After all, it feeds every other system, including the brain, skin, hormones, and thyroid. It also is key to iron absorption, weight loss, fertility, and inflammation reduction.

Because of differences in our gut microbiome and a host of other factors that affect the way our bodies respond to foods, simply copying a diet that seems to be working for someone else isn't guaranteed to balance your gut or resolve health problems. (We will take a deeper look at this in chapter 4.)

As a college student, I tried to use my eating habits and health goals to control my life, not knowing that those were the very things compounding to work against me. My steady diet of wheat crackers and presliced apples from a fast-food restaurant was destroying my metabolism one day at a time. The body needs energy to perform, and when mine wasn't getting the right kind in the right amount, it slowly paralyzed my digestion. While following a restricted diet worked at first, once my body caught on to these toxic behaviors, it shut down, and my regimen backfired. Not only was I not getting the full range of nutrients I needed, but I also wasn't feeling the safety needed to properly digest food. Such safety includes plenty of nourishing foods, emotional support, and healthy relationships and environments.

As I discovered, if the environment in your gut is out of whack, you won't experience the healing you're looking for. The gut must be in balance before anything else in your body can work at its best. And believe it or not, recognizing this is a huge piece of the puzzle for many people. Although what your microbiome requires to heal may be different from what someone else needs, certain principles of good nutrition are universal.

If you're tired of feeling sick and tired, keep reading. In the coming chapters, you will learn how to heal the innermost layer of the gut, known as the mucosal barrier, so that the good and bad can get to where they need to be in the body and you can see results . . . for *good*. You'll learn the principles of healthy nutrition that can lead to renewed freedom and health for your body, mind, and spirit. I hope you'll also come to better know God, the One who made you and promises to satisfy "your desires with good things so that your youth is renewed like the eagle's" (Psalm 103:5).

May you be kind to yourself, surrendering the temptation to reach for another diet pill, starve yourself, or overexercise to the point of exhaustion. May you be brave enough to stop cycling through fad diets, numbing with sugar and alcohol, and obsessively counting calories. May you trust that God gave you a body that knows how to heal itself when you take the time to trust it, fuel it well, and offer it healing. May you let go of any shame about habits that brought you here. As I tell my clients time and time again—we don't know what we don't know. Simply showing up and making small changes over time can lead to big results. On the other side of this deep work, you will be able to receive the truth that your body is a gift.

Tips for Tending to Your Gut

1. Avoid consuming chemicals used in the growing and processing of food by buying organic items, particularly produce that grows underground or from a plant without a protective peel or shell (such as carrots, strawberries, and potatoes).

2. When possible, select the freshest fruits and veggies over precut, prepackaged, and prefrozen ones. When preparing greens and veggies for packaging, processors generally use chlorinated water and other substances to help the produce last longer. Of course, purchasing and eating prepackaged spinach or lettuce is absolutely better than not eating either.

3. Pay attention to where your meat and eggs come from. What these animals are fed, you're eating too. If cows and chickens are eating soy and the beef and dairy industries are using synthetic hormones, then you're also consuming said soy and/or synthetic hormones.

4. Eliminate refined sugars. Stick to small quantities of real sugars, such as honey, maple syrup, raw cane sugar, and fruit.

digging deeper

1. How well would you say you have been listening to your gut? What is one way you might treat it better going forward?

2. While God created our bodies to know how to heal themselves, we cannot escape living in this fallen world. What is one health-related area in which you feel you've been fighting an uphill battle?

3. Are you ready to incorporate God's wisdom around food into your thinking and decision-making? If so, what thought or habit can you ask Him to help you with today?

4. Have you been tempted to continue trying the latest diets without considering what your body may need to truly heal? If so, take a few minutes to think and write about the underlying goal. Would meeting that objective lead to a short-term fix or to lasting health and freedom?

5. If you've ever experienced shame around food, consider writing about it. What would it feel like to invite God into that place and release that shame to Him while you work to address physical healing at the root?

THE NUTS AND BOLTS OF NUTRIENTS

HOW TO MAKE FOOD WORK FOR YOU

Let me tell you about the night that was by far one of the top three moments in my life. I came home around 10 p.m. carrying a bundle of flowers and immediately fell onto the floor with the kind of sigh I'd only ever heard in movies. I landed right outside my roommate Mallory's door. She was sitting on her bed working on her laptop with the door open—a perfect opportunity for me to thoroughly distract her. I couldn't speak—I was only capable of staring at the ceiling while stroking my colorful bouquet. Mallory watched, perplexed. She'd seen me leave earlier that evening for what I called a "casual" date with a guy I'd met only recently.

Her confusion turned to giggles, and she finally asked for details. "Mere! Tell me everything!" Because that's what girls do when one of them comes home from a date that has completely changed her life.

I had met Daniel on a blind date two weeks before. For our third date, he invited me to his place for dinner. While I enjoyed being with Daniel, who was kind and handsome, I wasn't expecting to be blown away that night—especially over the meal he prepared. As soon as I sat down in his kitchen, he popped the cap off a cold bottle of organic cream soda and set it down in front of me. Swoon. I couldn't believe he had remembered that on our first date I'd mentioned in passing that I enjoyed cream soda. Then as we relaxed in his dining room to the sound of classical chill music, he served a unique appetizer of roasted beets, candied pecans, mint leaves, and crushed pistachio. He then plated steak, orange-glazed roasted carrots, crispy duck-fat potatoes, and prosciutto-threaded peas for each of us. The dessert finale was a poached pear that had been soaking for hours in cinnamon apple juice as it baked in the oven.

"Mallory, Daniel and I eat the same way!" I told her as I described the evening. "I'm coming undone." By now, I was committed to eating gluten-free, dairy-free, and soy-free and knew it would be hard to find someone who not only followed that protocol but also cooked just about every meal from scratch that way.

"And you thought he was going to make chicken and veggies," Mallory said, laughing.

There was a moment of silence until I hesitantly asked, "Mal . . . ?"

"Yeah, Mere?"

"How do you know if you've found the one?" Within seconds, we were hanging off the side of Mallory's bed checking Google for every sign of being in love. As Mallory read each one off, I responded in my head: *Check. Check. Check.*

Lack of emotional support is as damaging to the mind and soul as the lack of a nutrient-rich diet is damaging to the body. I hadn't received the emotional support I needed, so I was caught off guard when God gifted me with the real thing through Daniel. Just as the soul needs the healthy love of others in order to heal and flourish, so the body requires real food and the right nutrients to heal.

After years of therapy and a healthy marriage, I no longer have to go online to be sure I'm in love with someone. Likewise, when I feel physically good in my body, I don't have to google to find out whether I am well: I just know that I am. That is the goal here. There's no exact formula to achieve physical health. In addition to following the guidelines in this book, be sure to check in regularly with yourself to ask, *How am I feeling?* As you learn to trust your body, you'll gain freedom.

When we don't eat nourishing foods, it can be difficult to fully connect ourselves to the tasks that God has appointed us to do while we are on this earth. The enemy does not want us to be free, and he often uses food—God's gift to fuel our bodies—as a way to hold us back.

God intended for you to pursue good health, and there is absolutely no shame in fighting for it. You can have the results that you want by accepting this holy invitation of deep healing. I'm going to teach you how to help your body do just that. Let's begin by looking at how eating nourishing foods has deeply spiritual impacts on healing both body and soul.

HOW GOOD DO YOU FEEL?

When I was skipping breakfast and eating a severely restrictive diet, my gut was slowly being destroyed. I was making it harder for my body to metabolize and use nutrients, not to mention more difficult to process the emotional pain I had endured in my past.

Signs of poor digestive health

While thankfully I didn't suffer from all the maladies below, I did experience some. It doesn't take many of these symptoms of poor digestive health to know you just aren't feeling or operating at your best:

- fatigue
- constipation/diarrhea
- bloating
- PMS
- hormone imbalance
- skin issues, such as adult acne
- low thyroid function
- depression or anxiety

- food sensitivities
- iron deficiency
- infertility
- nausea after eating
- candida
- parasites
- heartburn/reflux/GERD
- compromised immunity
- brain fog

Until it has been given time to heal, the body will not properly absorb nutrients. We don't intend to harm ourselves when we try new diets and consume foods that are considered healthy. But once the body signals that something is off (refer to the list above), it's important to pause and offer your body the space it needs to heal. When I allowed myself time for deep work with a therapist and a nutritionist, my body came into alignment and my soul found freedom. It was a both/and situation. By the time I met Daniel, I had recognized the signs of poor health and had been working on my physical health.

Signs of good digestive health

When you're ready, your body can receive healing if you fuel it properly. It's not a quick fix. Years of circumstances got you to where you are, so it's crucial to take the time to learn skills for maintaining a healthy body and soul. As you make progress, you'll begin to see signs of improving health:

- few or no PMS symptoms
- clear skin
- little to no abdominal discomfort
- mental clarity
- little stress or good stress management
- energy that lasts all day (no midafternoon crash)
- good nightly sleep (seven to nine hours)

- one to three bowel movements a day[1]
- regularly drinking half your body weight in ounces of water
- strong, healthy hair and nails
- lack of unwanted weight around the hips and thighs

The gut and the brain are so deeply connected that when I went through counseling and gave my body the real food it needed, all my systems could finally fire together. Counseling enhanced my nutrition journey, and my nutrition journey enhanced counseling. The stronger your gut, the better your chance of staying calm and navigating intense life experiences with equilibrium. The more you remain emotionally regulated and stable during stressful and out-of-control moments, the more balanced your digestive system and the more likely you'll see improvements in your overall health.

YOUR GUT GARDEN

As mentioned in chapter 2, what you eat and how well your body absorbs nutrients determine how optimally the gut sends signals elsewhere. It is essential to tend to the GI tract as it acts like the mother of the body, nourishing every other system.

We *need* the gut to be in balance in order to see healing and positive results. This is why caring for the gut is so important when addressing just about any ailment you may be up against. While your specific issue may not be directly located there, what you are dealing with is likely impacted by a system that is tied to the gut in some way. Remember the static in the phone connection? Let's work on getting better reception so you can heal and be well. You need to be well to show up well.

Imagine that your gut is a beautiful garden. It is the most wonderful complex part of the human body where cells and tissues are fertilized and watered and where beautiful bacteria (or flowers) can grow. Just like in any garden, there are also unwanted invaders—opportunistic bacteria (weeds).[2] The physical environment and your life experiences will determine the rate at which flowers and weeds grow there. We all have both, but just as with any garden, it's the ratio of flowers to weeds that matters. Everything that goes into your mouth is either good (nourishing) or bad (invasive) for your system. The goal is for your gut to have enough of the good stuff to fight off the bad.

For your gut to thrive, you'll want to encourage the good bacteria to grow and eliminate or contain the bad gut bugs, or opportunistic bacteria. The goal isn't to pull every weed imaginable—that's really hard to do and not necessary. The goal is for the weeds to be a nonissue because the good bacteria are so dominant.

There's no formula or perfect ratio—it all comes down to what is the optimal function for *you* and how you feel. If you want hard data on the health of your GI tract, you can see a specialist who may run tests. However, there are several ways to determine how well your gut is functioning without testing.

It's easy to blame certain foods and periods of starvation or indulgence for all your problems, but that does a major disservice to yourself. If you have an imbalanced gut garden and you haven't taken time to pull the weeds and plant the seeds, then you won't experience the healing you need. This means the mental hang-ups you potentially have about which foods are good and bad, even to the point of obsession, are likely doing you no good. How sad to think of all that lost time focusing on a made-up list of good and bad foods just because of what you saw on someone else's plate, when it could all boil down to addressing your gut terrain instead!

DOES YOUR GARDEN NEED TENDING?

The mucosal barrier is the innermost layer of the gut. Comprised of tissue, blood vessels, nerves, and muscle, it controls which nutrients are absorbed and which allergens and other toxins are kept out. Your gut has an entire population of bacteria called microbes that help keep that balance of bacteria in check. The good bacteria line the intestinal wall to act as bouncers and knock out the bad bacteria trying to get in. The mucosal barrier is constantly working hard to detect what is good and bad, which is exhausting enough—even more so if you are overworking it with harmful habits, such as the overconsumption of processed foods, refined sugars, alcohol, and/or caffeine; chronic stress or overexposure to toxins in the environment or beauty and household products; and regular consumption of foods to which your gut is sensitive. If the GI tract takes too many hits, it may develop a condition known as "leaky gut."

Imagine your gut wall to be solid and intact with one door that opens to let in the right stuff. If the bouncers are lining the wall day and night, watching for invaders, then it's easy to kick them out and send them on their way. It's just as easy when the good guys come along for the gut bouncers to open that one door and allow more good things to come in and flourish. Now imagine that same wall with a bunch of tiny holes, some of which not even the good bouncers/protectors can see. These tiny holes are created when the impact of the harmful habits mentioned previously are too much for the gut to handle. With that, the protectors are standing by the door, still proudly accepting the good guys, but there's confusion on how the bad guys are sneaking in—through those tiny holes, which no fad diet will fix. (You can try various trendy diets all year long, but if you are not sealing up those holes, then the bouncers remain confused and the holes can get even bigger.)

The body is smart and resilient, so if leaky gut does happen, the mucosal lining has a backup, which is the immune system. We are going to learn about this in depth in chapter 5. This is why it's imperative to tend to this system as well.

It's important to feel confident in the body that God gave you and to fully invite yourself into your own life. How you show up, how you feel, and the memories you long for your future self to make depend on the way you nourish your body today.

WHY SHOULD YOU CARE?

Eating foods that nourish the body has a deeply spiritual impact. God gave us human bodies with physical needs for a reason. They are not only hosts for the Holy Spirit; they are necessary to participate in abundant life on earth. It's important to name your desire for health and believe that it's okay to work toward physical goals of all kinds, without the fear of becoming legalistic or obsessive. You can have a physical goal without feeling apologetic about it.

God intends that we care for our bodies so we can fully devote ourselves to the tasks He has appointed for us. We are commanded to love God with absolutely every part of our being—heart, soul, and mind—and to love others as ourselves (Matthew 22:37-40). Taking charge of our health is one way we equip ourselves to be "Christ's ambassadors" on earth (2 Corinthians 5:20).

What if, instead of subscribing to the new monthly diet that has hit the market with its flashy supplement subscription, we subscribe to the truth that God created our bodies to be good and to know how to heal themselves when they are working properly and are appropriately nourished? Though we are regularly exposed to external stressors and toxins, foods in their most real, God-given form help keep our bodies healthy.

By this point, you might be wondering just how food heals our bodies. First, when we learn how to properly prepare and consume nutrient-rich foods, we begin to fuel every one of our cells from the ground up. Through digestion, the food we eat is masterfully turned into new substances that have the ability to heal our bodies, clear our skin, grow our hair, balance our hormones, align our weight, and more. From the inside out, our cells are being fed, fueled, and multiplied—we are quite literally made up of the foods that we eat. This was how nourishment was intended.

Second, real food creates a robust stomach environment, which optimizes digestion—ensuring that nutrients get where they're needed. We strengthen our bodies so they can fully reap the benefits of the nutritious foods we are consuming. Eventually, we can enjoy our favorite foods and say no to restrictions and fad diets for good.

THE ACID TEST

To have optimal digestion, the stomach must produce adequate amounts of acid. Picture this: If you were to remove the acid in your stomach and pour it on the floor, you'd want it to be strong enough to burn a hole through the carpet or tile. The pH scale runs from 0 to 14 (0 being the most acidic); the stomach needs to be around 1.5 to 2 (quite acidic) to digest well. Why? Stomach acid is your body's defense against the pathogens and infections you are exposed to daily. Fortunately, the good bacteria can withstand the acid, while the bad bugs cannot. Stomach acid also helps move food through the GI tract more efficiently, cutting down on unwanted symptoms like gas, bloating, belching, cramping, and abdominal pain.

Having low stomach acid, a condition known as hypochlorhydria, can cause a host of downstream issues in the gut, including

inefficiencies digesting protein, which provides the body
with amino acids like tryptophan that are necessary for
increased mood vitality and tissue creation; and
inability to effectively activate digestive enzymes to break
down food.

After the stomach burns and churns food, it sends it to the upper part of the small intestine for absorption and assimilation. With its lower acidity, the small intestine cannot break food particles down further, though enzymes and bile from the pancreas, liver, and gallbladder continue digestion.[3] At this point, undigested food particles are sent further downstream and potentially into the blood, causing issues and exacerbating "leaky gut."[4]

It's common for people to assume that symptoms like heartburn—caused by acid reflux or GERD (gastroesophageal reflux disease)—are a result of too much stomach acid. The quick fix is to take an acid blocker, which may offer short-term relief. However, if the heartburn and reflux are the result of too little acid, the blockers reduce the amount of acid the stomach secretes even more, making the problem worse.[5]

Heartburn and reflux may be symptoms of inflammation of the stomach lining caused by different stressors. When the gut is thick and healthy, the acid causes no discomfort. If the lining is inflamed, however, the acid causes those unwanted symptoms. Fortunately, you can use natural remedies to boost stomach acid (see tip on page 44).

THE IMPORTANCE OF PROBIOTICS

In addition to increasing stomach acid, you can improve your gut garden by consuming prebiotics and probiotics. Probiotics are live bacteria that increase the good gut bacteria, and prebiotics include fiber-rich foods that nourish probiotics.

For good health, the good bacteria in your gut should outperform the bad bacteria. That enables the GI tract to defend itself against invaders or pathogens. A healthy gut environment is not about avoiding all pathogens, invaders, toxic chemicals, and mental or emotional stress, but rather involves being strong enough to stand up and fight against them when necessary. One way to do this, in addition to eating foods that are rich in prebiotics and probiotics, is to consume a good probiotic supplement. I recommend you look for the following when choosing one:

- at least 10 billion CFUs[6]
- spore-based probiotics with an enteric coating, which will help prevent destruction by stomach acid[7]
- a guarantee from the manufacturer, either on the label or insert, that the product was tested and certified to contain the stated amount of live bacteria[8]

WATER WORKS

The unsung hero in all of our health concerns involves water. It's so simple, yet one of the most powerful tools for healing. Water is our main source of energy and is necessary for all bodily functions. It's used to break down food and then assimilate nutrients from cell to cell. Water is responsible for increasing our body's ability to absorb the nutrients that we get from food. It helps nourish our joint connections, allowing us to work out without pain. Water is also responsible for flushing out toxins from our system.[9]

You might already know that you "should" drink half your body weight in ounces of water per day, but you might not know why. Water helps regulate your hormones, blood, immune system, and digestive processes, and when you don't get enough, your body lacks the ability to perform necessary functions. While drinking an adequate amount of water is important, it's just as important to ensure that your body is absorbing it well.

This is where electrolytes come in. Electrolytes are minerals that, when absorbed in water, have a positive or negative electric charge. Your body uses them to help regulate chemical reactions and preserve the balance of fluids inside and outside your cells.[10] Aiming to drink half your body weight in ounces of water with adequate electrolytes will serve you better than drinking a gallon without the nutrients. You can get electrolytes by adding trace mineral drops, electrolyte powder, or unrefined pink sea salt to your water, as well as by drinking coconut water.

REAL FOOD, REAL RESULTS

Notice that you do not have to strive for a perfect gut environment. A high-functioning or optimal digestive tract just needs to be in balance for *you*. There are a few ways to discern what this means, but the main thing always comes back to how you *feel*. Are you beginning to have more energy or a more positive mood as you seek to bring balance to your body? Are you experiencing fewer digestive difficulties? Are your pants getting looser? If you want someone to walk through this journey with you, I recommend reaching out to a practitioner in your area for more support and further testing. It might be tempting to give up or give in, but remember that gardens don't become beautiful overnight.

You have the opportunity to love your body because it is a gift from God. He cares for you, and He gave you the responsibility to tend to the garden of your body and soul. So *stand up and fight*. Take back what is yours. A great way to learn to love your body is by nourishing it the way God intended. As you care for the body God has given you, you can rest knowing that it is beautiful—just the way He created it.

Tips for Cultivating a Healthy Gut Garden

1. Take a good probiotic to help restore the good gut bacteria and defend against the bad ones.
2. Eat prebiotic- and probiotic-rich foods like kombucha, kimchi, sauerkraut, and anything fermented or pickled, which can help nourish the gut and feed the good bacteria.

3. Avoid or limit common offenders such as gluten, refined sugar, conventional dairy, dairy alternatives (see pages 49–50), and soy.

4. Increase stomach acid by taking in bitters (e.g., dandelion root, radishes, bitter greens), dietary protein, apple cider vinegar, or lemon juice.

5. Stay hydrated in order to keep nutrients moving and to help eliminate toxins and unwanted bacteria.

digging deeper

1. What non-nutritious foods do you find yourself reaching for on a regular basis? What is so tempting about these foods to you?

2. What can you do today to become more at peace with food and surrender this struggle to God?

3. What is one behavior you might commit to in order to consume more nutrient-rich foods?

4. When it comes to your body, what can you give God glory for today as you strive for better health?

4

WHY QUICK FIXES
DON'T WORK

SAYING NO TO FAD DIETS FOR GOOD

Though I couldn't have articulated it back then, one of the reasons I left Kentucky for Texas was my desire to put a sizable boundary between myself and some people who seemed intent on controlling me. Looking back, however, I see that I was trying to bring control to my own chaotic life by placing strong restrictions around what and when I would eat. In other words, I had run away from one form of control only to take up another.

I would go many hours without eating, and when I did eat, it would be tiny portions of food I thought were nourishing but were anything but. Despite my fascination with food and nutrients, I had yet to learn how they affected my overall health—not just the way I looked.

In my attempt to control my chaotic life, I used food to try to make myself feel better. I understood a few food "rules" and decided to follow them in an attempt to get what I wanted. I also tried various strict diets that controlled what I ate. When I followed the paleo diet, I primarily consumed meat and veggies. I eliminated all sugar, grains, and dairy from my diet as I followed Whole30 time and time again. I dabbled in the autoimmune protocol (AIP), keto, juicing, and more. Each set of guidelines led me to eliminate isolated food groups from my diet, which meant I missed out on key nutrients at various times.

Even when I was "successful" at these games of control, however, I couldn't understand why these regimens seemed to work for everyone else but not for me. I assumed they must have it figured out in a way I didn't. It was extremely frustrating, particularly because not only would I follow these eating plans to a tee, but I would take them even further by avoiding meals altogether or certain food groups "just because." I became obsessed with what was on everyone else's plate as I tried to see what worked. I didn't care if I liked something or didn't; if I saw someone I considered "healthy" eating it, I made it part of my diet too.

As a result, I was severely deficient in nutrients because I was either not eating or I was eating a ton of the wrong stuff. I was consumed by the thought of food, even tempted by diet pills a couple of times. Fad diets intrigued me, though they usually seemed to backfire, not work at all, or make me completely miserable. Years of this caused more stress and even more shame. I assumed that I must just have a broken body. Only later did I learn that these diets never worked because they were never supposed to work indefinitely. Could they be tools for people to learn how to eat? Sure. Could they temporarily help people form healthy mindsets around food and health as they tried to clean up their diets? Yes!

If you're looking for lasting results, however, you need to eat in a way that brings some measure of healing to your body. This means working really hard to fight for alignment so that your body can absorb nutrients and eliminate toxins properly; your gut microbiome can be rebalanced; and you can commit to a lifestyle change.

One of the few bright spots as I cycled through various diets was my interaction with a Christian therapist. Our sessions were truly life-altering; in fact, they helped me realize that my behavior around food was getting in the way of my working through emotional barriers. They forced me to ask myself: Why was I exhausted, emotional, hungry, malnourished, slow, and anxious when I thought I was doing all the right things? I wouldn't say that I had an eating disorder, but I absolutely had a bad relationship with food and disordered thinking around how best to fuel my body.

Noting my less-than-ideal food habits, a friend of mine encouraged me to see a nutritionist during my first year in Houston. Once I started seeing him, suddenly everything seemed to click. My therapy sessions were enhanced; I slept through the night for the first time in years; my anxiety nearly ceased; I experienced actual joy; I was alert for my quiet times with God; and I had energy to exercise, plan meals, and cook.

What caught me off guard was how much better my life was after just a few months of eating in a way that nourished my body and soul. I went from buying fast and convenient meals at the grocery store or restaurants to buying my own food and cooking every meal. Doing all that food preparation felt like a full-time job at first, but I never gave up and I've never looked back. Choosing to prioritize nutrition was one of the best decisions of my life.

Discovering the right kind of nourishment was so instrumental that I've devoted my life to teaching others to do the same. That doesn't mean it is always easy. As empowered as I felt by the way nutrients were healing my body and enabling me to stay more connected to God, I still had to work through childhood trauma and process through years of stress that had resulted in high cortisol levels and inflammation. God, therapy, and nutrients changed the entire game for me. Once I understood the power of nutrients to address healing at the root, I was able to make permanent lifestyle changes that matched the way God had designed my body.

What I learned is this: Specific diets may serve a purpose when they're approached with intentionality, but as a general rule, there is no diet that will work for absolutely everyone 100 percent of the time. Most of these diets are designed to help people bridge the gap between a symptom and a lifestyle change. For example, someone who recognizes that their food cravings are due to a sugar addiction might follow Whole30 as a way to eliminate all sugar from their diet. The AIP diet can be helpful for those with an autoimmune disease. The paleo diet is great if you want to learn to eat as our ancestors ate. All have their purpose.

Many people tend to follow certain diets long term (or adopt them permanently). Not only is that unnecessary, but such diets are usually ineffective once their short-term purpose has been served. They are designed to teach you what is missing from your diet or to target a certain symptom—not to keep you at a target weight or forever eliminate digestive symptoms.

Weight loss and true healing take time. You won't achieve gut health by eliminating major food groups long term or by focusing on just one part of your digestive system. If you take acid blockers because you suffer from heartburn caused by acid reflux or GERD but jump right into an elimination diet, you're likely to have a harder time seeing results. Healing the upper GI tract by addressing the root of symptoms like heartburn is an essential precursor to any elimination diet or healing protocol. Balanced hormones depend on the proper absorption and elimination of nutrients, so you have to address digestion issues before the hormone problem can be addressed. These are two examples of times when fad diets will not work.

"I'LL TRY ANYTHING"

Because so many variables influence each person's gut terrain, it's a terrible mistake to look at what someone else is eating and assume you should do the same. You have no idea what their stress level is, how they ate the week before, what their childhood diet was like, whether they've experienced trauma of any kind, whether they've taken too many antibiotics, or whether refined carbs and processed foods have ruined their blood sugar levels.

The reality is that what is on someone else's plate might be good for them but not for you. It might be nourishing to their body or to their genetic predisposition but not to yours. Rather than getting hung up on specific foods, it's important to remember that until you are actively working to heal and bring balance to the gut, specific foods are less important than the overall good/bad balance of your gut garden.

In fact, some foods that are offered as "healthy alternatives" to the real thing may backfire. Consider dairy alternatives, for instance. If you swap real milk for nut and oat milks that are riddled with thickeners, gums, additives, chemicals, inflammatory ingredients, and lectins, have you really solved any problem by going "dairy-free"? Such alternatives usually end up making people feel even worse because the stomach wasn't made for them.

Of course, nut and oat milks have become very trendy in the last few years. What I've realized is that it's important to trust what you're feeling and what your body is telling you. Don't just follow something blindly because it sounds cool or because other people are doing it. If dairy is a no-go and dairy alternatives become popular, it doesn't mean it's what's right or what's best for the human body.

In fact, once you've brought healing to your gut, it's possible you'll be able to enjoy foods—like real, full-fat milk or sugar—that you have avoided for years. I've watched people go dairy-free but not feel better until their gut was healed. Only then could they enjoy properly sourced organic milk with no issues.

If you really cannot tolerate dairy or you want to enjoy a milk alternative while on a gut-healing protocol, choose brands that have two ingredients—nuts and water—*or* make your own. Take control of what goes into your body and be confident that you know how to build your own plate.

WHY THE RESULTS OF FAD DIETS NEVER LAST

Healing is holistic. The common thread among fad diets is that each primarily takes one part of the body into account and disregards everything else. It's great to cut out sugar and grains for Whole30; you're addressing the body's needs to retire the sugar addiction circuits, and you may possibly even lose a few pounds. But what you're not doing is addressing the underlying pathways that trigger your body's craving for sugar and resistance to dropping a few pounds. Is there a nutrient deficiency, or are the detoxification pathways impaired? Is there any unaddressed trauma that needs to be looked at? Knowing the physiological reason for a craving or weight plateau helps you determine how to address healing at the root.

Only when any underlying issues are addressed (not just sugar and fat loss) will you see lasting results from something like

Whole30. If you don't address your body as an interconnected system, you may see quick results, but it's likely that your body will go right back to where it was as soon as you discontinue the diet. You might have even made the underlying issue worse. This may be your first step onto the hamster wheel—because something "worked" and then you're frustrated when it stopped.

Another temptation is to try something like paleo or keto. You remove the foods that aren't permitted, but are you considering how well your digestive system is working? Are there any unwanted pathogens that have been able to grow as a result of undergoing chronic or unresolved stress or eating highly refined foods for years? Following the paleo and keto diet for a few months or years might bring some of the desired results, but if you're not creating balance in the gut microbiome and increasing your body's ability to digest and absorb nutrients and eliminate toxins, then the second you stop these diets, your body will likely respond as it did before and your efforts will backfire again. So the hamster wheel continues to spin.

Sound familiar? Let's ditch the fad diets for good, okay? There's no need to constantly stress about something that isn't going to work optimally. Plus, following a list of food rules with no end in sight sounds exhausting. What if I told you that once you offer yourself the space and pace to heal your gut, no food will be off-limits? Does that sound scary? Maybe it sounds liberating! After you have restored your gut health, every food in its purest form can be nourishing and enjoyed without guilt. Think ice cream made with organic vanilla bean, sea salt, full-fat cream and full-fat milk that comes from hormone-free, grass-fed cows, and maple syrup for sweetening. The main thing to remember is to source ingredients as close to the real plant or animal as possible to ensure they are nourishing.

GETTING OFF THE HAMSTER WHEEL FOR GOOD

This might be some of the best news ever—you do *not* need to starve yourself, binge eat, take a million supplements, eat at specific times, do intermittent fasts, or eliminate all your favorite foods to see results. It's possible to lose weight and reach your goals within a reasonable amount of time without compromising yourself and/or losing your soul in the process. It's possible to see results without ever following another fad diet again.

Instead of chasing trendy diets (and loving the look of green juice more than loving the actual taste of green juice itself), you'll want to find the root of stress in your body and focus on a holistic type of healing that allows your body to digest well so that you can absorb nutrients, eliminate toxins, and see the results you've been longing for.

Healing the gut is the first step to ensuring that every other system and pathway functions optimally. Whether your main concerns are hormonal or immune issues, acne, anxiety, depression, IBS (irritable bowel syndrome), mood disorders, chronic stress, or weight issues, addressing gut health will lead to significant improvement.

LETTING GO AND LETTING GOD

Fad diets are appealing because they promise quick results for anyone who faithfully follows the program. That's why the hardest part about getting off the hamster wheel of these diets may be investing the time and more difficult work of learning about and preparing the real foods God created to nourish our bodies. In a world of convenience foods and quick fixes, taking the time to source and assemble nutritious meals can seem overwhelming. Fad diets, on the other hand, generally come with a list of restrictions and guidelines that offer a sense of control that feels good. I don't blame you if you resonate with this. Life is hard, and a list of rules sounds good if you thrive on structure.

Reader, your body is not broken. It's beautiful and miraculous, and it's giving you permission every single day to either accept or deny the abundant life God offers. You don't have to follow a particular list of rules to accept the gift of abundance; in fact, it's yours today, even if your body needs healing. Healing is beautiful and miraculous in its own way—it's why I became a nutritional therapist: to show people (by God's grace) that healing holistically is powerful, both physically and spiritually.

My favorite and hardest times with God have been when I was in the deepest pits of grief over my own trauma and physical challenges. The struggle to work through past stress and relinquish control over my own body caused an immense amount of pain. Scripture doesn't sugarcoat life's difficulties, but it does offer hope:

> In this you rejoice, though now for a little while, if
> necessary, you have been grieved by various trials, so that
> the tested genuineness of your faith—more precious
> than gold that perishes though it is tested by fire—may
> be found to result in praise and glory and honor at the
> revelation of Jesus Christ. Though you have not seen
> him, you love him. Though you do not now see him, you
> believe in him and rejoice with joy that is inexpressible
> and filled with glory, obtaining the outcome of your faith,
> the salvation of your souls.
> 1 PETER 1:6-9, ESV

Refinement in our lives doesn't just happen. It takes trials that require work to overcome. It's hard and scary to work through issues that have caused us pain, but being willing to face them head-on is what leads to the most valuable refinement. Just as gold becomes pure and genuine when put into a fire, so your faith—having been put through suffering and trial—is made better when you choose the path of fighting for healing. The fire is not awesome for obvious reasons, but you are made better as a result of it. Likewise, your body begins to heal when you toss out everything in your pantry that doesn't work for you, cook most of your meals, and eat healthy dishes you never expected to enjoy.

I'm no longer afraid of pain, suffering, and grief because I realize how much better I know Jesus as a result of my personal journey toward spiritual healing. I'm no longer afraid of food or tempted by any kind of diet because I gave my body the time it needed to heal and come into balance spiritually and physically. My life will never be the same, and I've made it my mission to help other people find this freedom. Once I realized that fad diets are just that—fads that fade away—and truly started to eat in a way that brought me healing and nourishment without having to follow a list of rules that didn't consider my entire body, I became free in my thoughts and relationship with food.

It's true that the healing process takes longer for some people, who may even need to work with a practitioner. But for everyone, no matter what, it starts here—with these guidelines for good gut health. If you are interested in working with a nutrition professional who will start you on your own journey to wellness, it's good to reach out to someone who takes a root-cause, holistic approach and, ideally, is certified. Many will offer a variety of tests (like gut, hormone, thyroid, blood chemistry, etc.) to identify areas of stress in the body.

Tips for Getting Off the Hamster Wheel

1. Say no to fad diets by shifting your mindset to eat in a way that's nourishing to your body.
2. Clean out your pantry, getting rid of any item that isn't real and/or doesn't have real ingredients. If you can't pronounce some of the ingredients or there are more than five on any label, chances are the item contains fillers and is not real. Don't overlook low-calorie items that contain sugar substitutes; they are not real food either.
3. Clean your fridge of any dairy alternatives with ingredients beyond just nuts and water.
4. Make a trip to your grocery store with no agenda except to become familiar with new foods along the outer perimeter of the store. If you're feeling bold, try one new fruit and/or veggie a week.

digging deeper

1. Reflect on any fad diets you've followed. Consider the reasons you tried them. When do you find yourself most tempted to jump on a fad-diet hamster wheel? Are you typically driven to start one because you're trying to fill emotional needs or because you want to have a certain body by a certain time? How might a more thoughtful approach to pursuing better health serve you better?
2. As you consider cleaning out your pantry of nonfood items and replacing them with real food, what concerns do you have?

3. Do you find yourself trying to cope with the struggles and hardships of life by turning to food? Why or why not?
4. Have you considered the difference between striving for better health and losing weight? How would you distinguish between those two goals?

WORK THE (IMMUNE) SYSTEM

HOW TO SUPPORT YOUR INTERNAL DEFENDERS

One afternoon when I was in high school, my little sister and I were hanging out in our backyard practicing hitting softballs. I had played shortstop and second and third base for years. At the time, my sister was around seven or eight, so I thought I had a thing or two to teach her. (I was neither a star nor the worst player on any team I was on. Little did I know that my sister would go on to be a Division 1 athlete playing basketball at the University of Kentucky.) A few minutes into our practice, I was gearing up to show off my skills and preparing to hit the ultimate home run. I had the tightest grip on the bat, and the windup was just right. When the ball came my direction, I swung so hard that the momentum from the bat twirled my entire body around. I ended up missing the ball entirely and slamming the top of my foot with my bat. Despite the pain and embarrassment caused by nearly breaking the top of my foot, all was not lost: I finally got the crutches I had always wanted.

As an athlete, I was that girl who was always fascinated by supplements, medication, ACE bandages—and crutches. I carried a gigantic water bottle and sports drinks everywhere. As it turns out, relying on outside remedies like energy drinks impacted my gut and its resiliency over time. Thankfully, I grew out of that stage pretty quickly, but when I look back at my younger self, I can't help but giggle at the ridiculousness of it all.

While I might have thought I looked cool hobbling around on crutches, as soon as my nervous system registered the pain, my own body had begun doing most of the repair work on my foot, which quickly swelled up. That acute inflammation was my body's way of responding to the injury.

Though my focus back then was misplaced, I was right to be interested and concerned about attending to injuries and remaining fit. What I didn't realize then was how tightly connected my immune system is to my digestive health. In this chapter we'll take a closer look at how and why they're related, as well as the types of food that improve the body's immunity.

IMMUNITY MATTERS

Each of us is exposed to approximately sixty thousand germs, bacteria, and viruses per day that live in the air, water, soil, food, plants, animals, and humans.[1] Billions of immune cells throughout your body are constantly scanning to protect you from any and all kinds of invaders. When the immune system discerns a problem or an invader, it kicks into gear, starting the body's process of healing itself. Your body generates two different types of immune responses: innate and adaptive. The innate system is your body's primary defender, and it includes all the defenses you were born with.[2] Think of the physical barriers of your body, such as your skin, the good bacteria in your digestive system, mucous membranes in the intestinal linings, and stomach acid.

You also have adaptive immunity, which supports your innate response.[3] Our bodies were designed to adapt to certain pathogens rooted in our particular environment and lifestyle. For example, when we are exposed to certain germs, the immune system tags those invaders so that it recognizes and can fight them more quickly the next time they show up.

Anything unrecognizable to your system, such as a toxin, chemical, bacteria, or virus, is known as an antigen. Because it is foreign, these molecules set off an immune response, and your body begins to develop antibodies against it.[4] The immune system takes note and doesn't forget the immune-triggering antigen. The more times the same antigen enters, the more effective the immune system becomes at fighting against it.

However, if the immune system is worn down, deactivated, weak, or impaired by an unhealthy gut microbiome, it may identify healthy substances and even parts of your own body as antigens. Over time, an overactive immune system may lead to an autoimmune response and/or illness, which is what occurs when the body's immune system attacks organs like the stomach, thyroid, or colon. This may result in health issues such as ulcerative colitis, lupus, Hashimoto's thyroiditis, and more.[5] This response reminds me of a game of dodgeball. If you're throwing a ball from the back of the field to hit opponents and knock them out, you have to be careful not to hit your own teammate who may be in the ball's path. Because the game moves fast, hitting someone on your own team is not out of the question—that's why it's important to stay alert, robust, and fast. It's the same for your intestinal lining. It's important to help it stay strong and alert so it can protect itself while attacking invaders.

About 70 to 80 percent of your immune cells are located in the GI tract,[6] and they work with the cells in your intestinal lining to create harmony within your entire body. In fact, this connection impacts your health and ability (or inability) to see lasting results as you strive for better health.

In chapter 3, we looked at how the gut lining helps keep unwanted invaders out and good bacteria in. From the time you consume food to the time its waste products are eliminated, the food you eat never enters the rest of your body unless the intestinal (gut) lining has given it the go-ahead.[7] That's why it's so important to tend to the health of that intestinal lining, which is constantly scanning its internal environment for nutrients and invaders to figure out what to do with them. As you now know, this lining needs to remain sealed to be at its strongest.

Your gut's immune system borders the gut lining, and the cells in the gut lining barrier work together with the cells in your immune system. Two other key immune-supporting players in your GI tract are the lymphatic system and the liver. Together they work to help the body absorb nutrients and expel anything the body doesn't need.

Because the immune system is a second line of defense for your digestive system, two problems may arise if it constantly has to protect against particles that should have been taken care of in the gut lining. First, if your immune system is overworked, it may lose its ability to defend against viruses and pathogens. Alternatively, if the immune system is on high alert and overreacting to invaders, it can lead to autoimmunity and further inflammation. That's why it's essential that we zip up the lining of the GI tract so the relationship between the digestive system and immune system can remain healthy and intact. We don't want bad blood between the two. Pun intended.

INFLAMMATION: THE NEUTRALIZER

Inflammation is a key tool in your immune system's attempts to vanquish threats and bring about healing. (Remember my swollen foot?) The immune system activates this complex biological response to target and clear harmful stimuli such as pathogens and irritants, or to initiate repair in injured tissue. Acute inflammation is a good thing. It is intended to be a temporary response to an injury or when the body detects invaders that may damage cells. While you can see inflammation in a swollen ankle or black eye, your body also uses it to attempt to deal with foods that trigger the body or with stress that your nervous system can't tolerate.

Inflammation becomes a problem when it's chronic, wearing down the body's ability to defend itself. It also is the source of many health problems, including neurological disorders such as dementia that tend to develop later in life: "If the level of inflammation predicts neurological disorders, and excess body fat increases inflammation, obesity is a risk factor for brain disease."[8]

To keep from developing chronic inflammation, we must tend to the immune system, including a focus on healing our digestive systems. However, in today's world, food sensitivities, allergies, chronic stress, environmental exposures, seasonal allergies, and synthetic or processed foods all contribute to chronic, low-grade inflammation—often in ways that aren't immediately detectable but that may contribute to diseases like type 2 diabetes and autoimmune disorders. Because it's impossible to avoid all stressors, we must control inflammation through anti-inflammatory foods and nutrients, as well as stress management, appropriate rest, healthy relationships, regular exercise, and other healthy habits.

Our bodies need antioxidants in order to fight inflammation, and they rely on a healthy diet and lifestyle in order to keep inflammation from becoming chronic. Interestingly, obesity is an inflammatory disease. That inflammation is caused by an imbalance in the gut. That's why it makes sense to stop "blaming" our failed attempts to reverse obesity on weak willpower and instead pay more attention to the health of our digestive systems. Addressing this gut balance before attempting any kind of weight loss strategy is the missing key to any weight loss journey. There's simply no way around it.

Food's impact on inflammation

Processed foods contain refined sugar, alcohol, gluten, dairy, and/ or soy, all of which can contribute to inflammation—particularly in people with sensitivities to these substances—by fueling the proportion of bad bacteria in our gut. Eventually this can trigger our immune system to respond with chronic inflammation. When inflammation becomes chronic, we create a pathway for invaders such as pathogens, viruses, and allergens. That's yet another reason to avoid these trigger foods.

Again, after you remove common offenders, it's imperative to take measures to repair the lining of the mucosal barrier in the gut. Substituting processed snacks and meals with plant-based foods can calm inflammation. Certain foods, such as nuts, olive oil, fruits, and vegetables, contain antioxidants that also seem to reduce inflammation.[9] (See the Whole-Body Health Protocol, which begins on page 157.) Once healing has taken place, you may be able to eat these common offenders in limited quantities without undoing everything you've worked so hard to accomplish.

Stress's impact on inflammation

Stress also impacts the immune system and inflammation. Simply put, when you face chronic stress, whether due to mood, life, food, or sickness, your body is more likely to generate acute inflammatory responses, which can lead to chronic inflammation. Of course, stress—even chronic stress—can't always be avoided. How then can you support your immune system during difficult seasons?

Researchers at Washington University in St. Louis compared the stress response of parents who had a child with cancer—an obvious ongoing stressor—to those whose children were healthy overall. This enabled them to evaluate the impact of ongoing stressful situations on the immune system. As expected, the parents of cancer patients had greater inflammation and reduced immune capacity. However, they discovered that these negative immune responses could be mitigated through social connections and support from the community.[10]

Likewise, researchers studying the effects of loneliness determined that isolation can alter immune cells and weaken the vagus nerve's tone.[11] Positive interactions and connections with other people, on the other hand, strengthen the vagus nerve, helping the body transition from a stressed (sympathetic) state into a calm (parasympathetic) one. This also leads to a stronger immune system and less chronic inflammation. In his book *Cured*, Dr. Jeffrey Rediger notes that "we are *biologically built* for positive love and connection."[12]

OTHER WAYS TO TAME INFLAMMATION

Support your circadian rhythms

Genesis 1 tells us that God's first act during creation was to call for light. "God saw that the light was good, and he separated the light from the darkness. God called the light 'day,' and the darkness he called 'night.' And there was evening, and there was morning—the first day" (verses 4-5). He set the earth in a rhythmic motion, and later when He shaped and breathed life into man, God locked a biological rhythm into every cell of the human body as well.

Our bodies run on a twenty-four-hour cycle, or circadian rhythm. On a cellular level, everything that happens is rhythmic: Our nutrient absorption, metabolism, cellular maintenance, cell repair and division, and cell communication are some examples.[13] The Sleep Foundation explains, "Circadian rhythms are 24-hour cycles that are part of the body's internal clock, running in the background to carry out essential functions and processes. . . . Research is also revealing that circadian rhythms play an integral role in diverse aspects of physical and mental health."[14]

We all have a master clock in our brains known as the suprachiasmatic nucleus (SCN). This clock helps each individual system to regulate and stay on a rhythm as well as sync our bodies with the light and dark from the outside world.[15] The SCN is located in the hypothalamus, which houses all of our cues for hunger, metabolic rate, mood, stress management, temperature regulation, and more.[16] Because the hypothalamus is attached to the pituitary gland, the SCN is indirectly connected to this gland, which regulates stress, thyroid hormone production, and reproductive hormone production. The SCN also connects to the pineal gland, which produces melatonin for sleep.

Finally, the SCN is connected to our retinas (eyes), so when we see light and dark, the SCN sends signals throughout the body. When the SCN is reset by light, it resets every other system, including all our digestive and immune processes.[17] Much like the ocean, the tides roll in and out, but a disruption—powerful winds, pelting rain—causes chaos. The waves begin crashing against one another and creating disharmony along the shore. With time, as the environment calms down, the waves begin to hush and there-fore can go gently back to their rhythmic patterns that are peaceful.

This is what we want in our bodies. We want peaceful rhythms that contribute to good health. Sleep—along with diet and physi-cal activity—affects how well our circadian rhythms function, so let's now explore its impact on our overall health.

Prioritize quality sleep

Adults consistently need seven to nine hours of uninterrupted sleep a night.[18] (Of course, this is the ideal. New moms, first responders, and shift workers are among those regularly challenged to meet this goal. That means they must find ways to support their bodies through this.) For now, however, let's consider how quality sleep relates to metabolism and immune function.

Most people operate on a twenty-four-hour biological clock that aligns with the production of important hormones on a natu-ral light and dark cycle. This cycle and sleep work together to regulate digestion, hormones, and body temperature. When you sleep, your body works hard to repair cells, eliminate toxic debris, and strengthen the immune system. Without adequate sleep, these processes are negatively impacted.

YOUR METABOLISM ON SLEEP

Research shows that sleep deprivation and interruptions to the normal circadian rhythm have profound impacts on metabolism. For example, researchers from the University of Chicago found that a mere four days of insufficient sleep slows down the body's ability to process insulin.[19] Because insulin turns sugar and other foods into energy, when its production slows, the body is more prone to storing fat.

YOUR HORMONES ON SLEEP

Two hormones, cortisol and melatonin, naturally regulate your sleep-wake cycle. The body will produce more melatonin around sunset to prepare for sleep. That's why it's essential to support the body's natural production of melatonin by avoiding caffeine after 2 p.m. and bright overhead lights and man-made blue lights (electronic screens) in the evening. Checking your phone, watching TV, or reading on your iPad at night can reduce your body's natural melatonin production.

Giving your body adequate time to wind down and adopting a healthy nighttime routine can dramatically improve your health. Try wearing blue-light blocking glasses at night, find a soothing skincare routine to calm your nervous system, and consider taking evening supplements like magnesium that your body may need.

Because the production of melatonin is predicated on the body having enough serotonin, which is produced in the gut, microbiome imbalances can lead to lower production of melatonin.[20] That can cause a host of sleep issues—even insomnia. Quality sleep and balancing the gut, then, go hand in hand.

Just before the sun rises and you wake up, your body naturally begins to produce more cortisol, which is the hormone responsible for controlling stress throughout the day and the way your body processes food as fuel (using it as energy or storing it as fat). By eating within one hour of waking and stepping outside to take in some sun, you help your body regulate cortisol and align with your natural circadian rhythm.

YOUR IMMUNE SYSTEM ON SLEEP

Have you ever noticed that during a season when you're not getting adequate sleep, you are more prone to sickness? Or that when you take a vacation right after an extremely busy season, your body shuts down and you get the flu as soon as you arrive at your destination? There is a reason why this happens: "When a person is sleep-deprived, the immune system creates an excess of pro-inflammatory cytokines, resulting in . . . inflammation."[21]

To replenish your immune cells, your body needs adequate rest. In fact, most immune cells are produced while you're sleeping. Research shows that as you near "the end of a full night of sleep, immune cells migrate out of the blood and into the lymphoid organs, which is where viral pathogens often accumulate after entering the body."[22] You are exposed to toxins and pathogens daily, so it is essential that your lymphoid organs (which collect these toxins) are able to detox from them safely and effectively. When your immune defense is strong, your gut is more robust. At the same time, a healthy gut encourages strong immune cells to flourish once the body has created them during sleep.

It's pretty profound to consider how the Lord created our bodies to work according to His design. The natural rhythms of work and rest are essential for the health of our bodies and souls.

Accept love from God

Just as the body is an interconnected system, so each one of us is part of a larger community. We were not meant to be alone (Genesis 2:18). God placed us on this earth to love Him and love others (Matthew 22:37-40). He demonstrated His love for us when Christ laid down His life so that we can live. One of the ways we love well is doing all we can to nourish our bodies and manage stress effectively.

One of my favorite examples of God ushering in deep healing—mind, body, and soul—to someone is found in John 8. This is the story of a group of religious scholars and Pharisees outing a woman whom they'd caught in the act of adultery. They also saw this situation as an opportunity to trap Jesus, so they brought her to Him and declared that she deserved to be killed by stoning.

Imagine how this woman felt. She'd been brought before Jesus in the most humiliating and vulnerable state. It isn't clear whether she was forced or had chosen to be with the man (who wasn't targeted). Regardless, we understand enough about the nervous system to know that in her stressed state, her entire body was impacted.

Now imagine this woman standing next to Jesus at the front of the crowd. After the religious leaders expose her sin and demand her death, Jesus bends down to write in the dust with his finger. Though we don't know what He writes, I picture her relaxing a bit as He tenderly and humbly takes a moment to pause and reflect. Imagine the hush that falls over the crowd when He asks the ones without sin to throw the first stone. As the implications of His words sink in, I imagine the woman finally taking a deep breath and relaxing her shoulders. Then, when the last of her accusers drop their stones and walk away, Jesus asks her a rhetorical question: "Where are your accusers? Didn't even one of them condemn you?" (John 8:10, NLT). He puts her story back into her own hands, graciously telling her to sin no more and sending her on her way.

John Piper says it was God's way of saying, "I am reestablishing your holy life. . . . I have just put it on a new foundation: my grace."[23] Piper adds, "You have to have an experience of grace in your life before you can pursue not sinning. If you try to pursue not sinning without an experience of amazing grace . . . you get heartless misuses of the law."[24] From all we've learned about how God designed our bodies, it was almost as if He was giving her body a second chance by reestablishing her nervous system and stress response on a parasympathetic level. That was something she could not do on her own because none of us are wired that way. We need love and connection from God and others to be healed, not only physically, but mentally, emotionally, and spiritually.

That doesn't mean that the woman's life was instantly different or that all of her troubles, fears, and anxieties disappeared; it just means she'd been given a second chance. What she did with that was on her. Would she honor God with her choices or continue to be gripped by sin? Either way, she had the chance to grab hold of freedom and healing because of what Jesus did for her.

While the choices we make each day may not be as dramatic as the ones Jesus invited this woman to make, we, too, can honor our Creator by choosing to support the design He built into us. We've explored Jesus' generous offer to give us life in abundance while we are on earth, and part of that involves being tender toward how we feel in our bodies as we live as His ambassadors. Our healing—physical, mental, emotional, and spiritual—matters to God, so wherever you are today, trust that you, too, can have a second chance. In fact, you can have as many chances as you need because God's grace never ends (John 1:16). Let your heart be loved and your soul be carried as you treat your body with excellence and take Christ up on His offer of abundant life.

Tips for Strengthening the Gut-Immune Connection

1. Eat fermented foods such as kimchi, sauerkraut, kombucha, yogurt, and kefir. These are excellent sources of good bacteria to keep your gut in balance.
2. Talk with your health care professional about taking a prebiotic if your immune system seems to be very underactive and slow to respond. Alternatively, ensure

you're getting enough prebiotic-rich foods like fruits and vegetables, specifically onions, garlic, and tomatoes.

3. Exercise regularly to keep the blood and lymphatic drainage system flowing.

4. Limit your exposure to environmental toxins such as scented candles or wall plug-ins, cleaning supplies, and car air fresheners.

digging deeper

1. Many people assume the immune system exists only to help us fight illnesses. What did you learn in this chapter about the way it functions?

2. What clues do food sensitivities, allergies, and environmental exposures offer to a person about the strength of their immune response?

3. Which common food offenders do you want to limit?

4. If you or someone you love suffers from a chronic illness or has received an autoimmune diagnosis, in what ways might God work during recovery? How could you cooperate to bring improved health and healing?

6

ODD COUPLE

THE GUT-BRAIN CONNECTION

I was too embarrassed to tell people what was happening. There was no predicting when or where it might occur—in the shower or while blow-drying my hair, standing in line at a Fourth of July food truck celebration, lying by the pool, even during workouts. It happened so often that I started to recognize the warning signals my own body was giving me. When I started to feel lightheaded, nauseated, and clammy, I knew I was about to go down—literally—so I'd better sit or leave the room so others wouldn't see me pass out. These fainting episodes started at the end of high school, gradually increasing in severity as I entered my midtwenties.

After witnessing a few of these episodes in the gym, my personal trainer encouraged me to see a cardiologist. Because I was scared, I decided it would be best to face my fears and find out from the doctor how long I had left to live (not dramatic at all).

I was connected to a heart monitor for forty-five hours; ran on a treadmill while being connected to wires for forty-five minutes; and had several echocardiograms, blood and urine tests, and X-rays. In the end, I was diagnosed with vasovagal syncope, a condition in which the vagus nerve overreacts to certain triggers, causing the heart rate and blood pressure to suddenly drop. As a result, the person faints. The most common triggers are stress, pain, and heat. This malady is often harmless, but it's also incredibly inconvenient.

The Nervous System

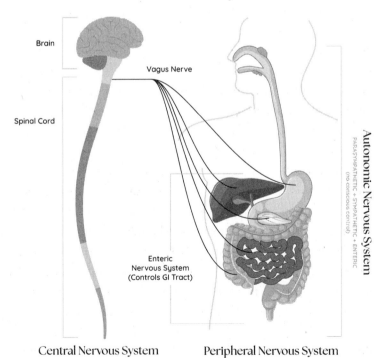

Brain

Vagus Nerve

Spinal Cord

Enteric
Nervous System
(Controls GI Tract)

Autonomic Nervous System
PARASYMPATHETIC + SYMPATHETIC + ENTERIC
(no conscious control)

Central Nervous System   Peripheral Nervous System

While you may not have this problem, you do have a vagus nerve, which is part of the autonomic nervous system. The nerve starts in your brain, runs down your spinal cord, and extends all the way into your gut. It is surrounded by a protective coating, called the myelin sheath, which is made of fatty tissue and enables messages to be sent quickly from the gut to the brain.

The vagus nerve helps your body exit fight-or-flight mode, which is controlled by the sympathetic (stress) nervous system, and return to a calm state under the direction of the parasympathetic nervous system. If the vagus nerve is suddenly activated, it may lead to fainting or gastroparesis, which is when food no longer moves into your intestines from your stomach.

When I was in the deepest pit of emotional pain, I had difficulty regulating my emotions. As you know by now, my eating habits didn't provide adequate nourishment. As a result, my body was under intense stress, which often triggered my vagus nerve to the point that I would pass out. In fact, the worse my situation became, the more I tried to control it with food, either by not eating or by exercising way too hard to get food out of my body fast. This cyclical pattern of behavior had negative impacts in both directions—on my mind and my body.

Addressing hurtful parts of my past by allowing Jesus (and a therapist) into my pain gave me power over those once-debilitating emotions. Hiring a nutritionist was another critical step toward learning how to treat both my mind and body well. I began sleeping better, experiencing less distress, having more energy, and enjoying my life again. How I fueled my body directly impacted my ability to show up for myself. What I later realized was that creating space for therapy, prayer, biblical community, and God's Word slowly began healing my undernourished gut as well. Over time the number of fainting spells decreased. I was experiencing true freedom in my body for the first time, and the people around me began telling me that they wanted the changes in their own lives that they saw in mine.

ALL ABOUT THE GUT-BRAIN CONNECTION

By the time you finish this chapter, I hope you better understand why what you eat directly affects how you mentally and emotionally show up for each day of your life. Even if you don't suffer from fainting episodes or gastroparesis, your gut-brain connection is still a powerful force that impacts how you feel in every aspect of life. This link is mediated by the autonomic nervous system, a network of nerves controlling involuntary functions of your body, like breathing and heart rate, that are critical for your survival.

Bear with me as we drill down a bit further into your nervous system—an unseen hero in your body that controls so many of its functions. Your autonomic nervous system, along with your brain, spinal cord, and sensory nerves, make up the overall nervous system.

The autonomic nervous system includes the sympathetic (fight-or-flight "stress" response) and the parasympathetic (rest-and-digest "calm" response). Its third component, the enteric nervous system, is the intestinal branch.

The enteric nervous system is responsible for controlling immune function as well as "blood flow, hormone release, and motility (the movement of food through the digestive tract)."[1] It's known as the "second brain" because it relies on more than thirty neurotransmitters that are also found in the central nervous system (which includes the brain and spinal cord) that control how we think, learn, move, and feel. A few of them, including dopamine and serotonin, are sometimes called "happy hormones" because of their effect on our sense of well-being.

Because of the neurotransmitters that connect the gut and the brain, the GI tract is sensitive to emotions like anger, anxiety, depression, and excitement. About 95 percent of the body's serotonin and 50 percent of its dopamine are produced in the gut and sent to the brain.[2] Are you beginning to see why GI function (or dysfunction) can have such an incredible impact on a person's mood? Feeling nervous before a meeting or sensing a pit in your stomach when something goes wrong can be explained by the connection between the brain and the gut. This is why reducing stress or treating anxiety can dramatically improve GI symptoms.

ANIMAL PROTEIN AND MENTAL HEALTH

I think it's important to acknowledge that when someone is diagnosed with a mood disorder, medications are often one of the first interventions considered to boost the level of serotonin and other feel-good neurotransmitters. (Generally, these drugs are paired with therapy.) I believe they can have their place, particularly if you need help in processing trauma, grief, or extreme stress or if you are working to recalibrate your digestive system so it can produce more of these essential neurotransmitters once again.

In other words, while the nutrients you need to help your body create these happy hormones can come from food, I also believe it is okay to lean on intervention when you need it. In addition, I would never advise anyone to stop taking medication for a mood disorder without consulting their doctor. In some situations, medication is a critical piece of the treatment plan, and it can actually be a valuable tool as people work toward healing their gut.

Ultimately, medications treat symptoms rather than the root causes underlying feelings of sadness and anxiety, which is why, in many cases, a combination of medication, therapy, and properly prepared nutrients is best.

Just as poor nutrition, trauma, and stress can impact or even determine what's going on in your brain, so the brain has a direct impact on digestion;[3] in fact, it's where digestion begins. The moment you start thinking about your next meal, the gut produces gastric juices in preparation for breaking down the food you're about to consume. While this connection between the gut and the brain is automatic, the foods you choose to eat determine how well your digestive system and brain work together—and what your overall mood will be.

The body's ability to communicate via neurotransmitters requires a clear path to and from the brain and the gut. If the gut is compromised due to food sensitivities or crowded with unwanted bacteria, pathogens, fungal overgrowth, and parasites, it will have difficulty sending signals up the neurotransmitters' pathways to the brain, which can lead to diminished mental functioning as well as anxiety and depression.

In addition, proper neurotransmitter development depends on the balance of a person's gut bacteria.[4] An overgrowth of unwanted bacteria and too few good bacteria will hamper the development of these neurons. A weak vagal nerve will struggle to use neurotransmitters to send messages related to digestion along the spinal cord to the esophagus and the gut. This results in undigested food sitting in the stomach, causing symptoms like gas, bloating, and constipation. Whether someone has an overtriggered vagus nerve or an overactive nervous system, it's important to stimulate the vagus nerve and work to regulate the nervous system to promote good digestion and healing.

We want the connection between the brain and the gut to be top-notch, right? That means properly fueling the brain so we are cognitively alert and emotionally regulated. In previous chapters, we've talked about the importance of balancing the microbiome. Here are additional ways we can keep this pathway clear:

- fuel the brain and body with adequate protein
- ensure the brain gets sufficient amounts of high-quality fat
- nourish the myelin sheath that protects the vagus nerve
- regulate the nervous system

YOUR BRAIN ON PROTEIN

To function well, the brain requires adequate amounts of quality-sourced proteins, which initiate neurotransmitter activity in the brain. These internal messengers are made from amino acids, "small molecules that are the building blocks of proteins."[5] Adrenaline, noradrenaline, dopamine, serotonin, and endorphins are just some of the neurotransmitters responsible for regulating pain and/or helping us feel good, calm, and emotionally stable; and all of them are made from amino acids.

Where do amino acids come from? From the body *and* from food. Of the twenty-two amino acids used in human protein synthesis, eight or nine of them cannot be made by the body. We *have* to get them from food. The most high-quality, absorbable forms of amino acids are found in animal proteins. Inadequate amounts of these essential amino acids will impair production of neurotransmitters. Taking it a step further, even if the body consumes the protein it needs to make the remaining amino acids, it still may be unable to do so if digestive health is poor. It comes back to considering the digestive system's two primary functions:

Is it absorbing nutrients, specifically the proteins needed to make amino acids? Is the body eliminating toxins so that it can focus on producing the amino acids? Because we may not know the answers to these two questions definitively, it's always important to ensure the diet has adequate amounts of quality proteins.

Research shows that fueling the body with adequate amounts of good protein can dramatically improve your mental health.[6] Fueling your body with the right kinds of proteins can help reduce and eliminate anxiety, stress, panic attacks, and more. It can also help reduce symptoms of insomnia and depression.[7]

Good protein sources

When considering optimal protein sources, you'll want to consume plenty of animal proteins as they are the most bioavailable form of nutrients.[8] Look for meat, cheese, nuts, and seeds that are as real and as close to the source as possible.

Some of the best sources of protein include grass-fed beef, pork, lamb, bison, buffalo, and elk; organic, pasture-raised chicken, turkey, duck, and eggs; organic, full-fat, grass-fed dairy products such as cream, milk, and raw cheese. Nuts and seeds (preferably sprouted) are also good sources.

Other plant protein sources include beans, soy, and lentils, but they are mostly incomplete sources of protein, lacking vitamin B_{12}. As a result, they supply an inadequate amount of the nutrients the brain and body need to function well. They are also commonly hard to digest and are allergens for a lot of people. Though legumes are a source of protein, they are also inflammatory, contributing to the imbalance that we are wanting to correct.[9]

This list is not comprehensive, but it can be a relatively good place to start when considering how to fuel your brain. To get adequate amounts of protein, you'll want to eat 1 to 1.5 grams for every kilogram of body weight each day. For my clients, that generally works out to between 90 and 130 grams per day.

YOUR BRAIN ON FAT

Though they've often gotten a bad rap, healthy sources of good quality fats are critical for your health. Fats help control inflammation, balance mood, provide energy, assist with blood clotting, and improve cognitive function and focus. Good quality fats also fuel the myelin sheath, the protective layer around the nerve cells, to ensure better communication between organs.

There are some unhealthy fats that are not recommended for regular consumption, if at all. These fats, which include soybean oil and canola oil, have to be heavily processed as they are extracted from their source. This is not ideal since fats, like other nutrients, should be consumed in their purest form.

Good, healthy fat sources

- omega-3s: wild-caught fish and fish oils like salmon, cod, sardines, and anchovies; egg yolks and walnuts
- omega-6s: organic nuts and seeds like pumpkin and pistachios; cold-pressed oils from sesame, flaxseed, evening primrose, and black currant
- omega-9s: olives, avocados, almonds, hazelnuts, and macadamia nuts, along with cold-pressed oils from each of these
- certain saturated fats: coconut oil, fats from pasture-raised animals like beef, lamb, bison, buffalo, and pork

Unhealthy fat sources

- canola oil
- corn oil
- cottonseed oil
- palm oil
- safflower oil
- soybean oil
- sunflower seed oil
- vegetable oil

Keep in mind that most restaurants cook with unhealthy oils, which are relatively inexpensive and can be used in industrial machinery. When eating out, I am generally more interested in the cooking oil used than in a particular food. For example, potatoes are healthier if they are roasted with a dash of olive oil than if they are fried in bulk using canola or soybean oil.

YOUR BRAIN ON NUTRIENTS AND ACTIVITIES

Nutrients that help heal the nervous system

- B vitamins—These help produce neurotransmitters.
- Electrolytes—These serve as spark plugs for every system in the body, especially neurotransmitter function. They include sodium, potassium, magnesium, and calcium, among other trace minerals.
- GABA (gamma-aminobutyric acid)—GABA helps with relaxation; low levels can lead to anxiety. The body makes this amino acid, though fermented foods like pickled cucumbers or beets, kefir, and yogurt are also good sources.[10]

- Magnesium—This mineral helps the body to relax; also one of the first minerals to be depleted when the body is under stress. Supplementing and/or enjoying Epsom salt baths can be a good way to replenish magnesium and promote relaxation throughout the body.

Balancing your blood sugar and avoiding overconsumption of caffeine will also improve the way your nervous system functions.

Activities that help heal the vagus response
- cold plunges
- gargling and chewing
- exercise
- massage
- laughter
- prayer
- healthy relationships with others
- acupuncture
- relaxation

Activities that help regulate the nervous system
- listening to relaxing music
- walking outside in nature
- letting yourself cry, which is the body's way of expressing emotions in order to self-regulate[11]
- intentional breathing
- seven to nine hours of quality sleep at night
- co-regulation with a loved one or in therapy[12]
- exercise
- getting a massage

- journaling
- setting boundaries to create more energy for yourself and to protect your own emotions and ability to self-regulate
- any activity that promotes a calm state of being

GOD WANTS AN INVITATION

In addition to focusing on your physical and mental health, it's important to pay attention to your spiritual health. When I was in the midst of seeking healing for my mind, body, and soul, I remember being afraid to ask God to join me in the depths. After all, I wasn't sure what was deep down inside me, and I didn't want to disappoint Him more than I felt I already had. I also assumed that God would be disappointed in me for wanting to work on my physical health instead of focusing on more "holy" and spiritual matters. Prior to seeing a nutritionist, my only concept of "working on myself" and "eating healthy" had not been all that healthy. Frankly, I'd been chasing the wrong things in the wrong way. I wouldn't eat because I wanted to be skinny to gain others' approval.

My counselor once told me that "nothing will change until the pain of remaining the same becomes greater than the pain of change." With that, I decided to stop resisting and invite God into my journey.

Reframing my view of my God-given body around the truth that it is a gift from Him helped me to slowly start to believe that it was okay to want to shed extra weight. I was taking care of myself so that I wouldn't miss out on the blessings and memory-making moments He wanted to give me.

One cold winter morning not long after I moved to Houston, I got up before both of my roommates while the house was still dark. As I walked through our kitchen, the only sounds breaking into the quiet of early morning were our creaking wood floors and coffee brewing, gently splashing against the glass pot. After pouring myself a cup and adding creamer for the perfect blend of morning goodness, I slowly made my way to the couch, where I anticipated a long time of study, prayer, and reading Scripture. Once I sat down and covered myself in my favorite white blanket, I opened my Bible.

I was surprised by what happened next. Unexpected tears fell on the open pages on my lap, leading me straight to the feet of Jesus. In that moment I finally believed that God wasn't reluctant to meet with me and everything I had to bring to the table—my emotions, my past, my health, and my relationships.

Even though I couldn't pray in that moment, I stopped trying to claw my way up and out of being uncomfortable and truly felt at peace with my pain. Beginning that day and continuing several days afterward, I would show up and let Jesus be with me while I cried. It was probably weeks before I was physically able to read any words on the pages of my Bible again, yet somehow in the silence, as I trusted that God was safe enough to invite to join me, a spiritual transaction occurred. I let down my walls, took deep breath after deep breath, and felt the knots in my stomach start to untangle. The control I had long fought for was lifted.

The shame I had felt about my desire to work on my body was about to change as well. After I had asked God to walk with me through the depths of my past and heal open wounds, I invited Him to heal my body. That meant giving up control, trusting my nutritionist, finding a workout routine that I deeply enjoyed, and no longer skipping meals.

I took to heart the apostle Paul's words: "We demolish arguments and every pretension that sets itself up against the knowledge of God, and we take captive every thought to make it obedient to Christ" (2 Corinthians 10:5). *The Message* puts it like this:

> The world is unprincipled. It's dog-eat-dog out there!
> The world doesn't fight fair. But we don't live or fight our
> battles that way—never have and never will. The tools of
> our trade aren't for marketing or manipulation, but they
> are for demolishing that entire massively corrupt culture.
> We use our powerful God-tools for smashing warped
> philosophies, tearing down barriers erected against the
> truth of God, fitting every loose thought and emotion
> and impulse into the structure of life shaped by Christ.
> Our tools are ready at hand for clearing the ground of
> every obstruction and building lives of obedience into
> maturity.
>
> 2 CORINTHIANS 10:3-6

In order to take something captive, it's helpful to identify where it came from. Returning to digestive health as an example, if you are chronically bloated or constipated, figuring out what is driving that symptom will be crucial to correct it. Relying on a laxative won't steer your body to what it needs to heal itself in the way God designed it to do. Likewise, trying to distract yourself with hours of TV won't eliminate recurring negative thoughts. Instead, taking your thoughts captive is a God-given way for you to regulate your mind. Not only will it give you a foundation of truth where you can line up your thoughts with God's, but it will give you space to breathe deeply and experience a full-body freedom and healing.

Your thoughts and attitudes—good or bad—originate somewhere. Recognizing their source is essential in allowing God to bring healing. Exposing the roots of your sadness, anxiety, or depression gives God a chance to meet you there and minister deeply to your soul, revealing any lies you believe. He takes your sadness and gives you Himself. Processing emotions with God's help will boost your efforts to regulate the nervous system just as healing the gut can address digestive issues.

This kind of deep work takes time, and it may even feel painful at first. Yet only when you choose to no longer mask the symptoms will you be freed to enjoy life abundantly. Just as it can take weeks, months, and years in therapy to overcome emotional trauma, so it can take your body that much time to heal as well. There's no exact formula for everyone, which means it may take longer for you than for someone else. Regardless, remember that you are not irretrievably broken and that God cares about you and the body that He gave you.

As it turns out, God wired us with the *need* to tend to our physical bodies. He created our bodies with mucosal linings and neurotransmitters for a reason. It's not wrong to want to lose weight if our bodies need to lose fat. In that case, losing weight means we are going to show up as the best version of ourselves. It's not wrong to want to address chronic gut issues. We just need the tools to know how to honor the bodies that we've been given.

I experienced firsthand how God brings His healing self into our lives as we fight for our physical health, whether we are working to correct bad habits, addictive behaviors, poor attachment styles, trauma, unhealthy coping mechanisms, eating disorders, food woes, or a negative body image. Tending to my physical and emotional health only enhanced my spiritual healing journey—as I know it will do for you.

Tips for Brain and Mood Boosting

1. Be sure you're getting adequate animal protein and healthy fats in your diet.
2. Address inflammation in your body.
3. If you haven't already done so, begin taking a probiotic to increase good gut bugs.
4. Work to balance blood sugar by avoiding refined sugar, eating more fiber, and exercising regularly.

digging deeper

1. How might changing what or how you eat transform your mental health?
2. Which step toward developing a healthy gut-brain connection are you most interested in pursuing: fueling the body with adequate protein; fueling the brain with adequate good-quality fat; avoiding refined sugar; or balancing the microbiome? What is one step you can take today toward that goal?
3. If you have suffered—or are suffering—from depression or anxiety, what steps can you take to nurture your body?
4. What one activity to help regulate the nervous system (see pages 81–82) will you try this week?

7

STRESSED OUT

THE UNSEEN COSTS OF TOXINS AND STRESSORS ON YOUR BODY

One morning during my senior year of college, I woke up and saw a text alerting me that a loved one was missing. I immediately panicked; my chest tightened and my hands trembled as I tried to figure out what was going on. How should I respond? On the one hand, I was concerned for this person; on the other hand, I was hundreds of miles away, with final exams to take and a retail job to work that night. After expressing my concern and confusion in the text I sent back, I was told that if I didn't leave school to help with the search, I was unloving.

Because I didn't want to be seen as selfish and was addicted to trying to fix things, I left campus, missing my final exam and work shift that evening. When that day ended, I drove around in the middle of the night trying to find someone who didn't want to be found in the first place. While this escape artist tried to get distance in a dramatic way, I had no idea that I could set up any kind of healthy boundaries at all.

What I didn't realize then was how devastating unhealthy interpersonal dynamics and emotional stress were to my health. In my desperation to get some control over my life, I restricted my diet to those wheat crackers and apples and engaged in vigorous exercise. Both—in combination with stress—were destroying my metabolism. To properly digest food, your body needs safety—and that looks like nourishing foods, emotional support, and healthy relationships and environments.

I'd soon learn that the things I was doing to try to pull myself together—both in my body and my soul—were just leading me deeper into a cyclical trap of toxicity. My restricted diet worked at first because it was new, but once my body caught on to these toxic behaviors and continued to feel unsafe, it shut down and my regimen backfired. I now know those efforts would never bring lasting results or give me true freedom. This discovery can make a big difference in your life too.

HOW DOES A GUT BECOME "TOXIC"?

A healed gut is one that works for you and not against you. It cooperates with the rest of your body to identify and expel toxins. As we discussed in chapter 3, blaming certain foods, restrictive eating, or overindulgence is counterproductive. Obsessing about which foods are good and bad may do you no good if your gut is a wreck and your detoxification pathways have been compromised. At this point, it's likely that your body is recirculating rather than expelling unwanted toxins.

The good news is this: A healed gut can open these detoxification pathways so toxins can be pushed out. Although you can't avoid all stress, a healed gut can most likely withstand the stresses and toxins you can't avoid. It will offer you digestive freedom by functioning optimally and being an effective bouncer, drawing on strong detoxification pathways. At that point, the key will be to keep your system healthy rather than allowing bad habits (and stressors) to creep back in.

Before we talk about how to make that healing happen, let's consider what stressors and toxins we want to eliminate.

WHAT IS THERE TO STRESS OVER?

I define toxins as anything that adds stress to and harms the body—be they substances such as food additives like artificial colors and flavors or emotional drains like unhealthy relationships. Several types of external stressors increase our overall toxic load. They include processed food, refined sugar, environmental toxins like chemicals or heavy metals, antibiotics, toxic beauty products, alcohol, pharmaceutical prescriptions, and over-the-counter medications.

To get a sense of how these stressors affect your body, imagine an empty bucket that you start to fill with water. You want the water to remain contained inside, probably around the mid-fill line, so that the bucket will be manageable and easy to carry. Now imagine that your body is like that bucket, and each exposure to a different stressor adds another cup of water to the container. Once it is full, the bumps of life will cause it to overflow and make a mess. This accumulation of stressors is what we call our overall toxic load.[1] Everyone has a different sized bucket, largely determined by their genetics. (Food sensitivities, allergies, and insomnia are just a few possible signs of toxic overload.) This analogy helps explain why some people have a lower threshold for stress than others—and why some children easily get sick while some senior adults are robust.

You have always been exposed to stress, and you always will be. Still, it's important to be aware of those stressors so you can control what you can. As an example, if you are in a stressful season due to a life transition, relationship turmoil, or a hectic work schedule, it will be more important than ever to follow a healthy diet, avoid taking unnecessary antibiotics or medications, and forgo the cookies and alcohol at the party. On the other hand, if you are in a peaceful season of life, you'll have more freedom to enjoy a glass of wine with friends or stay up late to watch a movie. In addition, look at your stress bucket from the perspective of an entire day or season rather than an isolated meal. If you are served take-out pizza at your niece's birthday party, then work to support your body afterward. These are all examples of how to keep the stressors at the mid-fill line in order to reduce your overall toxic load.

WHAT EXTERNAL STRESSORS ARE MAKING YOU TOXIC?

Think your gut might need tending to, but you're not sure? Here are some signs and symptoms to watch out for: bloating, frequent stomachaches, constipation, gas, diarrhea, chronic UTIs, chronic or acute eczema flare-ups, dramatic mood swings, menstrual issues, infertility, anemia, high cholesterol, and an inability to lose weight.

Since toxins are anything that is stressful to the gut, there are far more stressors than we can unpack in this chapter. However, I want to touch on some of the most common gut-health offenders that, when properly addressed, will make the greatest difference to the most people.

Sugar

Fruits and vegetables contain appropriate amounts of sugar in its purest form, along with other nutrients that help break down those sugars. As a result, they cause few—if any—problems. These real sugars have little to no impact on blood sugar regulation, which is why they are permitted in small quantities on the Whole-Body Health Protocol (see page 157).

Refined sugar, however, is a different story. Unfortunately, if you pay attention to ingredient labels in the grocery store, you've noticed that just about everything contains some kind of sugar. No wonder, then, that the average American consumes about sixty pounds of added sugar a year![2] The most offensive ones are refined sugars found in products like breads, cookies, cakes, packaged foods, and candies. Not all sugar is created equal: The closer you get to the original—the sugarcane plant—the better it will serve your body. Nonetheless, sugar is sugar and does metabolize similarly. During the Whole-Body Health Protocol, you will eliminate sugar to help soothe and unburden your GI tract, but that doesn't mean you'll have to eliminate it entirely for the rest of your life.

WHERE DOES SUGAR COME FROM?

Sugar added to other food comes from a plant called sugarcane. Around AD 500, farmers learned that they could crystalize the sugar by running it through cycles of heating and cooling. This is how we got raw cane sugar. Processing techniques have developed since then, and when raw sugar is stripped even further, its color changes from brown to white. Brown sugar is only marginally better than white, but the whiter the sugar, the more offensive it is to the gut. And the more it is processed, the cheaper it becomes. What was once a luxury item became a staple and eventually an addiction.

For example, it's recommended that women consume less than six teaspoons of sugar per day, but the average American woman consumes around fifteen teaspoons a day. That's nearly three times as much as what the body can even process.[3]

WHAT IS SUGAR DOING TO YOUR GUT?

Refined sugar (and unprocessed sweeteners like raw cane sugar and honey, if consumed in too large amounts) is one of the top offenders leading to unwanted bacterial overgrowth in the gut. That's because sugar actually feeds bad bacteria and suppresses the immune system. Eating too much sugar reminds me of what happens when you stand over a fishbowl to drop in a pinch of food. Just as the fish dash to the top of the bowl, when you eat sugar, those little bad gut bugs in your garden begin to feast. You're essentially saying, "Here, fishy, fishy! Keep destroying my insides." And those bacteria love it—the more you feed them, the longer they're going to stick around. These bad bacteria, along with fungi like candida and yeast, begin to make a cozy home for themselves and become even harder to eradicate. In addition, sugar inhibits the body's ability to produce the appropriate amount of gastric juices necessary to break down foods.[4]

When sugar is metabolized in the body, it has a direct impact on blood sugar and whether the glucose level in the blood spikes, crashes, or stays steady. Having a stable blood sugar level is crucial for so many health reasons. When it's out of whack, it also compromises gut function, hormone balance, the female's monthly cycle, the regulation and processing of stress, inflammatory activity, and the ability to process other nutrients, which can lead to certain nutritional deficiencies.

When someone eats large amounts of sugar, the brain begins to signal to the body that it needs sugar to burn as fuel. The more sugar consumed, the more intense the need for sugar becomes.[5] In addition, the body doesn't dip into fat stores for energy; instead, the brain just continues to crave sugar. That is why it's so difficult to beat sugar addiction merely by trying to limit intake. When you remove sugar completely, the body begins to draw from fat stores for energy, and the brain has time to process the fact that it really doesn't need sugar for fuel.

If you find yourself craving sugar—a pattern that you can't seem to beat—it's time to stop beating yourself up for being so attached to sugar and start looking at the root cause of the craving in the first place. Addiction isn't something you can snap your fingers and get over—sometimes it can happen cold turkey, but it often requires strategy, patience, and a healthy kind of endurance. In other words, the blame for your battle with sugar might not be all yours.

WHY GOING SUGAR-FREE IS NOT THE ANSWER

Artificial sweeteners lead to the same cravings, sensations, and addictions as the real thing. When you taste artificial sweeteners, your brain is still signaled to feed the sugar addiction. In addition, artificial sweeteners have been altered during processing, making it difficult for the gut to properly digest them.

Gluten

Gluten is a protein (different from animal protein) found in wheat, barley, and rye. When consumed, it stimulates the release of another type of protein called zonulin, particularly in those with gluten sensitivity. An inflammatory protein located on the lining of the small intestine, zonulin is triggered by bad bacteria. It is an important defender against threats like food poisoning since it acts quickly to get those harmful bacteria out of the body. However, because it breaks tight junctions within the intestine, high levels also contribute to leaky gut, allowing undigested food particles into the bloodstream. It weakens the immune response in the GI tract, which is why some people who consume gluten experience reactions like stuffiness, headaches, bloating, and more.[6]

While not everyone is sensitive to gluten, I highly recommend eliminating gluten entirely from your diet when working on a healing protocol because it triggers the same foundational responses in everyone. It also stimulates a heightened immune response, which is the backup system to the gut. (For a reminder about the role of the body's immune response, see chapter 5.)

I am often asked why gluten seems to be less tolerated today when people could handle it hundreds of years ago. The answer lies in how it has been modified. In short, wheat is a grass made up of select proteins that, when grown in the wild, has a higher protein and nutrient content than wheat grown for commercial use. Through the years, food growers altered growing processes to increase production. In particular, nitrates and phosphates were combined to fertilize crops. This, along with new technology, allowed wheat to be mass-produced at a higher rate. One side effect has been an increase in the strength of the gluten in the wheat, making it more offensive to the human digestive tract.

A lot of the bread you see on store shelves today lacks nutrients because so many of the original ones have been stripped away while synthetic ingredients (including lab-produced vitamins and minerals to replace those removed during processing) have been added. The immune system recognizes these wheat-like substances as a type of invader, which eventually may lead to an intolerance or imbalanced gut.[7]

WHY GOING GLUTEN-FREE IS NOT THE ANSWER

Have you ever picked up a package of gluten-free cookies, crackers, or bread from the grocery store and investigated its ingredients? It was probably hard to interpret anything on the list. That's because when something is gluten-free, the gluten has often been replaced with processed ingredients such as fake sugars, gums, thickeners, and grains, many of which are hard to digest. That's why I never recommend choosing "gluten-free" items on a regular basis—especially during a healing protocol. Every now and then it may be less offensive than the real thing, but if you eat it daily, or even multiple times a day, you are contributing to a clogged gut.

STAYING HYDRATED

Water is essential for nourishing the body. It's responsible for moving nutrients from cell to cell and flushing out what the body doesn't need/use. As mentioned in chapter 3, your body needs electrolytes to absorb water. You can drink a gallon of water a day and remain dehydrated if your body is not getting the minerals/electrolytes it needs or if it isn't absorbing them. Think you might be dehydrated? Here are a few signs and related conditions: asthma, allergies, constipation, hypertension, type 2 diabetes, autoimmune diseases, heartburn, lower back pain, colitis, headaches, joint pain, and fibromyalgic pains.[8]

Follow these guidelines to ensure your body gets the water it needs:

- Drink water between meals.
- Consume water when thirsty.
- As soon as you wake up, drink sixteen ounces of mineralized water (containing electrolyte sources like unrefined pink sea salt or a dash of coconut water).

- For every eight ounces of caffeine you consume, drink an additional twelve ounces of water.
- Do not rely on juices, soda, coffee, or caffeinated teas for your water consumption.

OTHER TOXINS AND STRESSORS

Food can be a big contributor when it comes to an imbalanced gut terrain, but the presence of stress—including toxic environments, relationships, and behaviors in your life—can also wreak havoc internally. The neurotransmitters connected from your brain to your gut need a clear pathway in order to serve you well. Stress can block the path. (For a reminder about neurotransmitters and why they matter, see chapter 6.)

Emotional stress

Digestion begins in the brain, and if your mind is consumed with stressful thoughts, your body may go into fight-or-flight mode, which slows digestion. If chronic or acute stress is a regular part of your life and you are experiencing any kind of digestive issue, it's important to learn techniques that will help ease that stress so that your brain and your gut can return to a calm state that promotes optimal digestion.

The World Health Organization defines stress as "a state of worry or mental tension caused by a difficult situation. Stress is a natural human response that prompts us to address challenges and threats in our lives."[9] This can look like being busy at work, running kids to and from school and other activities, traveling, handling tension or a breakup in a relationship, eating foods that are triggering to the gut, changing jobs, moving, getting married, getting caught in traffic, being exposed to environmental toxins and chemicals in beauty products. . . . Sounds like we are up against a lot, right? Well, we are.

Experiencing stress of any kind—especially in large amounts—leads the body to release cortisol, which contributes to inflammation. This inflammatory activity can disrupt the gut microbiome and allow opportunistic bacteria to grow. Once digestion is impaired and the wall of the gut has been compromised, undigested food particles have an open invitation into the bloodstream. This in turn activates the immune system. Because it doesn't recognize undigested foods, the immune system responds as if they were invaders. It releases cytokines and histamine into the blood, which inhibits the body's ability to break down fat. In fact, cytokines signal the liver to release more fat and sugar into the blood, resulting in the body storing more fat.[10] Eventually, this chronic immune activation results in inflammation that makes losing weight very hard, even when doing "all the right things."

Because cortisol contributes to inflammation and is released in moments of stress, it is crucial to address and learn to manage stress on any healing protocol. Of course, it's tempting to reach for a block of chocolate when you're stressed. However, by consistently looking to food as a reward or a bribe, you may unintentionally lead the central reward system in the brain to develop an obsession around food that interferes with your overall health and desire to see results. That's one reason I'm cautious about the term *self-care* when applied to food as treats or rewards. I love food, and I love how food can touch a deep part of that pleasure center in the brain. Food can be a fantastic source of celebration, but it's dangerous when consistently used to cope on hard days.

At the end of a long, stressful day, it's far healthier to spend time relaxing with your friends or spouse, taking a walk outside, calling a long-distance friend, or taking a long, hot bath. Other ways of coping with stress could include any combination of the following:

- walking after breakfast to help regulate the body's natural rhythm of cortisol
- creating a consistent nighttime routine that includes putting away all screens and drinking hot tea, both of which encourage your body to wind down and prepare for a night of deep restorative sleep
- sitting in a sauna for ten to thirty minutes daily to release stressors and toxins through sweating
- getting a massage
- listening to spa music in a dark room, without using your phone or tablet
- engaging in yoga, Pilates, or another form of light exercise
- praying or keeping a gratitude journal

Boundary issues

God wired us for connection (see Genesis 2:18). We weren't meant to do life alone. Our early connections and attachments are crucial for our sense of security, as well as how we see the world and make decisions.

As a teen and young adult, my desire to preserve unhealthy relationships led to a lack of interpersonal boundaries. I didn't want to be selfish; I wanted to be the peacekeeper. I kept a smile on my face, even as I allowed others to control me at the expense of my schooling, work responsibilities, and mental health. My decision as a college senior to drop everything to meet someone else's expectations is just one example of how I let others control my actions in an unhealthy way.

Healthy boundaries are an essential part of our overall health.

Naming what we will allow and not allow is just like reinforcing the mucosal barrier that lines the gut to protect it from harm. We need to draw an invisible line around ourselves so we can welcome in the people and influences that have a positive impact on us and keep out the behaviors that lead to chaos. Of course, there is a delicate balance between giving up on people or situations too soon and protecting ourselves from harmful people or situations that prevent deep healing inside us.

Licensed therapist Nedra Glover Tawwab defines boundaries as "expectations and needs that help you feel safe and comfortable in your relationships."[11] Just as our bodies need to feel safe to digest well, we need to be emotionally safe in order to thrive in relationships. When relationships feel chaotic and emotionally unsafe, the body recognizes this tension, which directly affects our physical health. When the body holds on to stress, a cascade of events can result, including weight gain, insomnia, disease, autoimmunity, infertility, digestive issues, and so much more.

Along with shedding stress from our toxic exposure to foods, products, and our environments, we also must shed unhealthy or toxic behaviors. Sometimes this looks like creating new boundaries so that once-unhealthy relationships have the opportunity to thrive; at other times, it may look like closing the chapter on certain relationships/friendships completely.

As believers, our ultimate security comes through Christ (Romans 8:1; 1 Corinthians 6:17), yet we also seek safety and security through healthy relationships on earth. To feel safe, we must be able to say the word *no*. This isn't a bad word, and using it doesn't make us selfish. It's the way we give ourselves a voice and stand up for what makes us feel secure.

According to Dr. Henry Cloud and Dr. John Townsend, we may not say no because we fear hurting someone's feelings, being abandoned or punished, or being viewed as unspiritual or selfish.[12] Yet saying no can be expressed in respectful ways: "I disagree," "no, thank you," "not right now," "I will not," or "please stop." When we fail to exercise our right to say no when we know we should, unhealthy boundaries begin to creep in. People may start to use and abuse us, walk all over us, manipulate us, gaslight us, blackmail us, and cause an immense amount of stress.

ADDRESSING EMOTIONAL STRESSORS

Establish boundaries

Once you've assessed the relationships in your life and realize that you need to create boundaries in your relationships, it will be crucial to communicate your needs and then uphold your end of the deal. You want to be kind, but you also want others to know that you expect them to respect your boundaries and needs. While people who truly love and care for you will work with you to honor these limits, don't be surprised if you receive pushback or defensiveness from "toxic" people. The changes you begin to implement to make your life healthier and safer may not sit well with them.

Though it may be difficult, here are a few things you can do to hold boundaries:

- Stop agreeing to do things you do not want to do or that make you uncomfortable.
- Let people know how you feel when they do, act, or say certain things to you.
- Resist the temptation to feel selfish when you clearly define your needs.

- Avoid talking *about* someone who has offended you and begin talking directly *to* them (see Matthew 18:15; Ephesians 4:29).
- Refuse to assume anything about someone else's actions.
- Stop feeling responsible for how others might feel when you communicate a healthy need of your own. Their reactions are their responsibilities.[13]

One of the hardest things for me in setting firm boundaries was becoming brave enough to state them. I was so used to relating in a certain way that I was afraid to shake things up. I feared the loss of the relationship. I feared being isolated if someone rejected my needs. It took me nearly a decade to shape and uphold boundaries with a family member I loved because it was so hard. I longed for the relationship to mend itself; I didn't want to come across as selfish or rude by having "rules." In the end, regardless of being told time and time again that I was self-centered and unloving toward them (and everyone else), I knew that putting up an invisible fence was the only way to begin addressing codependency, enmeshment, harsh words, and overwhelming chronic stress.

So how do you develop healthy boundaries?

- Clearly communicate your needs. This can be so hard if you're not used to doing this. You are responsible for setting and communicating boundaries; what others do with them (and how they feel about them) is ultimately on them.

- Don't feel the need to overly communicate or satisfy everyone else's curiosity. You're allowed to need something without having to justify it or explain it to others.

THE (GOOD) FOOD SOLUTION

- Be consistent in your requests.[14] I once had a counselor who explained it to me like this: When you repeatedly tell a child not to jump on their bed and they finally understand it, you will have to start over if you allow them to jump on the bed even once. Much like a child won't understand why you made an exception when they jumped on their bed, people will not understand why you don't always stick to your boundaries. That's why if you make a request, you must stick to it—even when it gets difficult.

Be willing to let go

I want to encourage you today to allow God to meet you exactly where you are and to help you let go of anything that is getting in the way of a healthy mind, body, and soul:

> Do you see what this means—all these pioneers who blazed the way, all these veterans cheering us on? It means we'd better get on with it. Strip down, start running—and never quit! No extra spiritual fat, no parasitic sins. Keep your eyes on *Jesus*, who both began and finished this race we're in. Study how he did it. Because he never lost sight of where he was headed—that exhilarating finish in and with God— he could put up with anything along the way: Cross, shame, whatever. And now he's *there*, in the place of honor, right alongside God. When you find yourselves flagging in your faith, go over that story again, item by item, that long litany of hostility he plowed through. *That* will shoot adrenaline into your souls!
>
> HEBREWS 12:1-3, MSG, EMPHASIS IN ORIGINAL

Did you spot the references to "spiritual fat" and "parasitic sins"? If you have allowed these inside you, it's time to get rid of them. In addition to a gut reset, it may mean revisiting unhealthy relationships and addressing any underlying stress in your life. Healing in your body won't happen in isolation from your mental and spiritual healing—they go together, always.

At this point, you may feel devastated that you've been "missing something" for much of your life. You might be tempted to feel shame for the ways in which you've mistreated your body through the years, whether in the name of "good health" and "seeing results" or because food seemed to be the only place you could turn for comfort. Maybe you feel bad for allowing your gut garden to get out of control so that you've potentially lost years of food freedom and physical healing.

Listen: You didn't know what you didn't know, but it's never too late. I pray this book will encourage you and give you hope that wherever you are today is the perfect place to start allowing your body to heal and your habits to change. If you're discouraged, I've got incredible news for you: Your gut is extremely resilient, and you can bring your gut garden back into balance through healthy changes to your diet, lifestyle, and environment. God made us with bodies that are strong enough to heal, seal, and repair themselves, even after years of damage. It may not be something that happens overnight, but I bet it will happen sooner than you think.

We live in a fallen world, so we will be exposed to sin and external stressors until we meet Jesus face-to-face. Still, God intends for your body and your faith to be made whole. As you work to recenter your gut, it will be essential to recenter your heart deep in the truths that God speaks over you. Because you are made in the image of God (Genesis 1:27) and God is love (1 John 4:16), each day can lead you one step closer to your sanctification and renewal in Christ Jesus.

Tips for Reducing Toxic Exposure

1. Eliminate or cut back on items on the "Foods to Avoid" list (see pages 190–191).
2. Invest in a good water filter and then stay properly hydrated.
3. Find ways to reduce stress by engaging in quiet activities that soothe the soul, like reading a good book, journaling, or taking a yoga class.
4. Surround yourself with friendly, encouraging people who build you up rather than bring you down.
5. Enjoy ten to thirty minutes in an infrared blanket or sauna to help promote sweat.

digging deeper

1. In what ways can you be more disciplined when it comes to what you put into your body and how you handle environmental toxins?
2. How can you set firmer boundaries with yourself and others in order to eliminate toxic stress in your life?
3. Are you often tempted to use food to self-soothe after a hard day? What healthier forms of comfort might you turn to instead?
4. What is one thing about the healing power of food that you've learned in this chapter?

8

THE MISSING LINK

THE TOLL TRAUMA TAKES ON YOUR HEALTH

I began working with Jackie after meeting her at one of my speaking engagements. She had struggled with stomach pain, nausea, cramping, constipation, diarrhea, and occasional bouts of vomiting for nearly eighteen years. She had low energy but intense cravings for sugar and caffeine. After three months of working with me on her nutrition and other health habits, Jackie reported significant improvement. She had much less stomach pain, though it hadn't disappeared entirely. Because she had gained new tools through our work and had become more mindful of her food and lifestyle choices, she felt confident that she could continue her healing journey on her own.

A year later, Jackie reached out to me again. Despite doing everything we had discussed, she hadn't seen much more improvement. She struggled with the thought that she was broken or that God's plan didn't include healing her body and ending her pain. We prayed together and discussed how stress and trauma can block physical healing. I recommended that she also meet with a licensed professional counselor to begin dealing with any emotional pain.

After running some tests to identify the specific strains of bacteria in her GI tract, we made some minimal adjustments to her food choices, supplements, and lifestyle. She also met weekly with her therapist, which enabled her to work through some past traumatic events and unhealthy relationships. Within five months her stomach pain and cravings were gone. I'll never forget the moment she told me that she was experiencing a new level of freedom. She was nearly in tears as she described how the hard work she'd put in had resulted in her feeling truly healthy and energetic for the first time in nearly two decades.

I've spent countless hours working with clients like Jackie on planning meals, choosing supplements, and developing exercise plans, only to come up against one of the most important barriers to healing—unresolved trauma.

Our bodies hold on to the unprocessed events we experience. The resulting thoughts, feelings, and emotions are first captured in our brains and then felt throughout our entire bodies, even if we do not recognize this happening. The body is so smart, and there is constant communication between systems. The brain, gut, and immune system signal back and forth all day long. When something happens to us that is traumatic or too much to process at once, the body prioritizes survival, activating the flight-or-fight response while holding on to our pain until the body feels safe enough to deal with it. Just as we learned that our bodies need to be in a parasympathetic state to optimally digest food, the same is true of our emotions. Our minds cannot process them until it feels safe to do so.

Emma reached out to me a few years ago specifically for support surrounding her depression. She knew there was a link between the brain and the gut, but she didn't quite know what it was. She had been working with a therapist for a while, but she also wanted to address her depression by healing her body. We were able to work together to create a customized plan that included food, supplements, and lifestyle changes. Within eight months, she reported feeling full of hope and joy for the first time in years.

After years of working with clients and researching food and nutrients, I'm convinced that people's inability to lose weight and heal their guts is often connected to damage done to their nervous systems by past trauma. I think it's one of the most important and under-discussed topics surrounding weight and related health issues. Now you might be tempted to skip this chapter if you assume you can't relate or if you're uneasy about considering your past. I understand that from my own experience: Some experiences are flat-out hard to revisit. Let me encourage you, though, that if you can stick with me through this chapter, you may well discover the missing link.

ATTACHMENT AND HOW WE CONNECT WITH GOD

Research shows that trauma survivors suffer more illnesses than other people. In fact, "survivors of childhood trauma are some 5,000 percent more likely to use drugs, attempt suicide, and suffer an eating disorder."[1]

God designed us with an innate need and desire for connection, and getting this core need met is critical to our health and longevity. From the day we are born, the way we relate to others determines how our bodies experience, process, and release stress. From infancy, the way we connect with our primary and secondary caregivers determines how we navigate the world around us. It also directly affects our later ability to meet any health goal, including weight loss, improved immune or hormone regulation, or fertility.

In the 1950s, British psychologist John Bowlby began developing the concept of attachment theory, which suggests that infants are biologically programmed to develop attachments with others as a means of survival.[2] Obviously, this need begins from the moment we take our first breath. Infants depend on their caregivers to feed, clothe, and change them. They also rely on their parents or caregivers to provide the soothing needed to regulate their systems—both emotional and physical.

Attachment Cycle

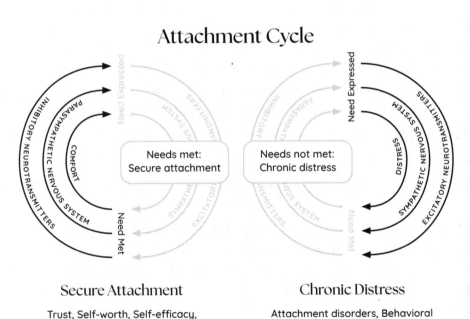

Secure Attachment

Trust, Self-worth, Self-efficacy,
Self-regulation, Mental health

Chronic Distress

Attachment disorders, Behavioral
dysregulation, Mental illness

Ideally infants learn early on that safety is provided by one or more particular individuals. As infants feel and express their needs, their bodies are stressed and distressed, and a ton of excitatory neurotransmitters fire in their bodies. This happens hundreds of times a day for little ones. When an adult picks them up, cradles them, feeds them, and lovingly touches them, their needs are met and they are comforted. This enables their bodies to return to parasympathetic mode, and their neurotransmitters to calm down and send appropriate signals again. These babies learn what secure attachment feels like. They learn to trust that their needs will be addressed, which gives them self-worth and self-esteem. Over time they also learn how to regulate themselves by becoming strong and healthfully independent, knowing their world is safe to explore. They can navigate difficulty and return to parasympathetic control relatively easily.[3]

Of course, for a variety of reasons, a baby's needs won't be met every single time, even by attentive caregivers. When a baby's needs are frequently unaddressed, however, the child is left in a state of chronic distress. Their neurotransmitters are constantly firing, cortisol is being released, and they're not able to get their nervous system back into a parasympathetic state. This is extremely hard on babies who do not yet know how to regulate themselves, resulting in attachment disorders, behavioral dysregulation, and even mental illnesses.

Mary Ainsworth, a colleague of John Bowlby, took his information one step further by conducting experiments designed to measure babies' reactions when their mothers exited and then returned to a room. She and two other researchers eventually identified four distinct patterns of attachment and how they manifested early in life.

Secure attachment: Children who have caregivers they can trust to meet their needs in a timely manner are upset when separated from their caregiver and joyful when they return. These children know that their caregivers, while not perfect, are reliable overall.

Insecure attachment (avoidant): Children who learn they cannot depend on their caregivers exhibit no or minimal stress upon separation and reunification with their caregiver. They may even avoid or ignore caregivers when they return.

Insecure attachment (ambivalent/anxious): Children who learn that their caregivers are unreliable show greater levels of distress upon being separated and reunited with their caregiver.

Insecure attachment (disorganized): Children who suffer abuse or neglect exhibit no predictable pattern of attachment.[4]

While these patterns describe their effect on children only, the attachment style we develop as children carries into adulthood. Psychiatrist Curt Thompson summarizes the effect of each attachment style like this:

- Secure children　　⟵⟶　　Free adults[5]

Free adults (secure): They are able to build healthy, strong, enduring relationships. As children, they felt safe, heard, seen, and understood, even if things were not perfect.[6]

- Insecure-avoidant children Dismissing adults

Dismissing adults (avoidant): They often fail to build long-term relationships because of their inability to engage in intimate behavior—both physically and emotionally. Whether their childhood caregivers were neglectful or simply busy, adults with this attachment style tend to keep people at a distance and may lack emotional empathy.

- Insecure-ambivalent/anxious children Preoccupied adults

Preoccupied adults (ambivalent/anxious): They often fear rejection and abandonment, and they show codependent tendencies. They find it difficult to rely on themselves for emotional regulation because they received inconsistent caregiving.

- Insecure-disorganized children  Adults with unresolved trauma or loss

Adults with unresolved trauma or loss (disorganized): They struggle to trust others, and their behavior is inconsistent and unreliable. Caregivers were often their source of both comfort and fear. Adults with disorganized attachment often endured trauma, abuse, or neglect as children.

When someone grows up with unmet needs, abuse, or trauma, they remain on high alert. As we've learned, this nervous system state impacts not only their emotional state, but how well the gut, immune system, and neurotransmitters send (or don't send) important messages throughout the body.

Trauma and unmet needs—even if suffered years before—continue to have a silent impact on your current physical health and your success in meeting health goals. Trauma and insecure attachments don't just leave the body; they need safe permission in order to do so.

TRAUMA/STRESS AND THE NERVOUS SYSTEM

When faced with an experience that threatens your survival or a pain that you can't process in the moment, your nervous system takes control and carries you through the situation. God designed this fight-or-flight system to take over long enough so that you can get through the difficulty and then process it later. Whether you're being chased by a bear, driving a car you notice is about to be struck, or having a difficult conversation with a family member, your nervous system instantaneously responds. Once triggered, your brain's hypothalamus activates the pituitary gland (located at the base of the brain) and adrenal glands (sitting on top of the kidneys). Your muscles tense, and hormones like cortisol and epinephrine are released into your bloodstream so you can respond immediately to the threat. Once the event has passed, the body has to use up those hormones to get back to a state of calm. Quality sleep, exercise, deep breathing exercises, and laughter all help keep cortisol levels in check.[7]

The effects of stress and trauma vary from person to person—even two people who've lived through the same events. How you perceive an experience determines how your body will react to it and how effective your body will be at processing and eliminating the stress hormones. We can define trauma, therefore, not as an event, but as the result of the way in which a person experiences that event.

THE SEEN AND UNSEEN TOLL TRAUMA TAKES

Despite repeated attempts at eating real foods and beginning new workout routines, Emily remained overweight. She was convinced that God was punishing her. When she came to me, she was also losing her hair, not sleeping, and experiencing significant anxiety. When we dug into her diet and health history, it looked as if she was doing "all the right things." However, with a combination of talk therapy and a gut-healing protocol that was unique to her, she started seeing results within a couple of months. Just over a year later, not only did she feel good in her skin, but she was no longer blaming God for a broken body. She had needed the right tools to support her body, which made it feel safe enough to respond. I led her to the right spot, but then she did the hard work.

If you've believed for years that your body is broken, I wish I could hold your face in my hands and remind you that your body is, in fact, beautiful, not broken. If you've endured mistreatment at the hands of others or were never taught how to self-regulate or healthfully attach to God and those around you, it's not your fault. If chronic stress is unaddressed, it could result in a blocked pathway from the brain to the gut. That makes it difficult for the body to clean things up and clear things out. You don't have to trace every traumatic/stressful event back to your home of origin. Perhaps you endured one particularly traumatic event when you felt your life was threatened or a chronic series of traumatic/stressful events—things like constantly moving, changing jobs, navigating troubled relationships, or being made fun of.

While I care about addressing stress and trauma because of my own experience, I'm also passionate about it because researchers have identified childhood trauma as a major risk factor for obesity and the development of eating disorders in adults. People who experienced insecure attachments as children and never processed them as adults have been on such high alert throughout their lives that they may not even have the self-esteem or motivation to care about their bodies. This is an entirely different set of issues to work through because motivation and drive are big parts of allowing the body the space it needs to heal.

Unfortunately, one way we've learned to try to self-medicate as a means of coping with trauma is by not taking care of the body well, whether through substance abuse, isolation, alcohol abuse, or abuse of food. In my work with clients, I've discovered that many people who've experienced trauma overeat. These are just some of the reasons:

- It gives us a sense of self-control.
- Indulging is a way of seeking self-pleasure.
- It numbs the pain from unresolved trauma that's too overwhelming to address.
- We lack understanding of how our bodies work.
- We aren't motivated to care about our health.

I don't blame anyone for any of this because—like I've said—life is so hard. That's why trauma and attachment work can be so profound for those who long for healing in their bodies but who have no idea where to look except to food and/or fad diets. Going deeper can often be the missing link.

You know the saying "Time heals all wounds." That's fake news. Intentionality, proper nourishment, and believing that God loves you, has always been with you, and wants the best for your life—even during all the painful events—are what allow healing to happen.

In a TEDx talk, Dr. Robert K. Ross explains that people with three or more exposures to childhood traumatic events see their health decline faster in adulthood than other people.[8] In addition, some of the top causes of death, which include diabetes, heart disease, stroke, homicide, suicide, and liver disease, can often be linked to trauma.[9]

I experienced a lot of trauma and stress during my teens and early twenties that I was unable to process, so my body held on to the effects of my experiences without me even realizing it. I lived in a chronic state of fight-or-flight for years, which led to poor digestion, imbalanced hormones, weight gain, and more. I was under so much stress that my body would randomly shut down by passing out—hence the vasovagal syncope diagnosis I describe in chapter 6. My body needed to learn the skills to enter into a calm state, reducing cortisol production so that my body felt safe enough to heal.

The most powerful and purposeful parts of my healing journey included conversations with safe people and intentional prayer. As I began to share the deepest parts of my story in counseling— the parts I wished would always remain buried—healing began to happen. At that point, I had difficulty emotionally regulating myself on my own. I hadn't grown up with the skills—I had to be taught. I learned ways to calm my body, whether by going on a long walk, taking a bath, exercising, getting a manicure, shutting off my phone, talking with a therapist, or sitting in a sauna. Such activities actively reduce cortisol and move stress out of the body, whether or not we are conscious of it.

Another great tool I discovered is grounding, a means of connecting to the present moment. Walking barefoot outside is one powerful form of this practice, which reconnects us with God's creation. Though it might sound a little "out there," it's been clinically proven that grounding "stabilizes the physiology at the deepest levels, reduces inflammation, pain, and stress, improves blood flow, energy, and sleep, and generates greater well-being."[10]

As I discovered—and research confirms—we can be taught how to self-regulate when tended to by another person who listens to us, holds us, or processes our pain with us. This is why therapy is an effective tool: Just being able to share your story and pain as another person (whether present physically or in a safe virtual environment) acknowledges you and your history is enough to begin to build the secure attachment you might have missed out on as a child. Therapy can also provide a relationship transference in a safe environment; in other words, you can finally achieve secure attachment to someone who responds to your pain and helps you process past trauma. God redeems all things, even unhealthy attachment. Your childhood does not determine your adulthood in the eyes of the Lord. Your adulthood is heavily influenced by your childhood, but it's not determined.

If you are hurting today, I pray that you would find a friend who will graciously hold your grief with you and not judge you or tell you to hurry up and climb out of it. A friend who pours you some hot tea and hears the pieces of your broken heart and lets you share as much or as little as you want with zero expectations. Then I pray that if you have considered therapy, you will have the courage to seek someone to walk with you through your pain on a deeper level.

SAFETY EQUALS CONNECTION

One of the best decisions you can make is to allow God to be a part of your healing process by inviting Him into the depths of your life and recognizing any false beliefs you hold about Him. In other words, you may discover that you've transferred the attachment style you developed with your parents or other primary caregivers to God.

People learn to filter and view God through whatever lens they've experienced growing up. If they had an insecure attachment to their caregiver, they likely view God as unpredictable, insensitive, and uncaring. Trusting God and allowing Him into their lives may be difficult.

Such fear and insecurity is as old as time. When Eve succumbed to temptation in the Garden of Eden, she ended up in a state of stress and shame. But rather than further shaming her and Adam, who ate after her, God the Father covered their vulnerable and naked bodies. He demonstrated deep love despite their shame and mistakes. This helped them return to parasympathetic living. They *needed* God, someone outside of themselves, to help them regulate that unfamiliar sense of deep shame.

Even when human connection is frail and broken, God still cares and is there for you. To put it plainly, He is the healer and redeemer of your nervous system, the safest place for you to begin living in a parasympathetic state. That reality is not meant to shame the caregivers in your life or place the blame elsewhere. Most likely, the people who were chosen to give you life and care for you during your vulnerable years genuinely did the best they could. We will never know how their own attachment styles affected them, but we can usually assume that even if their best and most loving was not much, it still was that—their best—and we need to recognize this, even if it means loving them from a distance.

Learning to release any blame and separate yourself from the sins of others is a great place to start regaining healthy connections, repairing chronic sympathetic nervous system dysfunction, and healing the heart and soul. Doing so while also working on healing the gut, immune system, and gut-brain connection will bring emotional and physical results that will allow you to finally participate in the abundant life God offers.

Tips for Supporting a Healthy Nervous System and Attachment Style

1. Fuel the brain with adequate amounts of protein and omega-3s.
2. Explore somatic therapy relief techniques to help process any residual pain/trauma impacting nervous system function.[11]
3. Ask God to lead you to a safe friend or therapist with whom you can begin to share your story and struggles.
4. Practice grounding (see page 116) as a way to begin to connect to the present moment.

—digging deeper—

1. What areas of unresolved trauma in your life need to be addressed? If you are unsure, do you have any eating habits (overeating, forgetting to eat) that may point to underlying trauma or pain?
2. Have you been in therapy and seen it through in its entirety? If not, what have you learned in this chapter

about why working with a good therapist might help you process trauma?

3. How might your attachment styles be interfering with your view of God and your desire for Him to be a part of both your emotional and physical healing?

4. How do you experience the truth that, whatever your past and attachment style, God deeply cares about you and longs to clothe you with dignity and to replace any shame you may feel?

9

SLOW DOWN

WHY STOPPING TO REST IS CRITICAL

In 2005 I spent a week in South Africa that changed the way I thought about food—and its connection to rest—for good. I was part of a church group working with a missionary who was helping plant a church in a rural village without electricity or running water. Our role was to go door-to-door, telling everyone about the new church launch. I visited more than fifty homes, and in each one I noticed families hard at work and always cooking. Meals were prepared over outdoor fires, and all the water was drawn from a well several miles away. On our last day there, a local family invited a few of us to take part in their daily routine. They wanted to connect and to lavish us with their hospitality.

We met them at their home early one morning just before sunrise. Our first task was to gather fruit and vegetables from the fields. We walked for what seemed like miles to search for potatoes, beans, and beets. Meanwhile, the men spent the day procuring and killing a goat for meat. While they spent hours skinning, prepping, sanitizing, and cooking the goat over an open fire, the women and children prepared all the side dishes. We spent hours peeling and boiling the beets and potatoes. We walked nearly an hour to the well in order to draw pots of water. By the time we had collected the water and started the long journey back to their home, I could only plod along, exhausted. The native teenagers, on the other hand, steadied fifteen-pound buckets of water on their heads and giggled as they walked. This was when my entire perspective shifted. It hit me that this was their way of life, day in and day out. And they appeared genuinely to be having a blast during every phase of this meal preparation.

We returned to their immaculate home with its packed-dirt floor and one wooden table. In addition to filling the cooking pots, we filled two large basins with water. One would be used to wash the dirty dishes; the second for rinsing them. Once the beets were boiled, one of the women showed me how to mash them with a kitchen tool that resembled a large wooden pestle. Another woman tended the fire; still others kept rotating the side dishes so all would cook evenly.

By 6 p.m., dinner was nearly ready. The table was set with mismatched dishes, silverware, and napkins, and it was one of the most stunning sights I've ever seen. Then we spent two to three hours consuming that meal. It was one of the longest, most beautiful days of my entire life.

Something soul-shaping happened to me that evening. That was the first time I realized that some parts of the world don't even understand the concept of fast or convenient foods. Our hosts didn't have ovens they could set to 350 degrees and walk away from for an hour. Instead they worked hard each day to prepare a meal that would nourish their entire family, with enough leftovers to snack on the next day (assuming they could be preserved and served without refrigerators or microwaves). For them, preparing food meant making sure the fire didn't burn out, rotating dishes so they were thoroughly cooked, and trying to prevent anything from going wrong because if it did, *they had no backup.*

YOUR BODY WILL NOT DIGEST UNTIL YOU REST

What I didn't realize until I began studying nutrition was the necessary connection between good digestion and rest. The South Africans I shadowed embodied one way to prepare real food and then savor it with others. However, we don't have to move to another country or get rid of our modern conveniences to spend unhurried time with our families. We can be thankful for electricity and our working refrigerators and stoves, which speed up or eliminate many backbreaking, labor-intensive chores. But learning to slow down will take time and effort—especially because we are used to breakneck living and eating.

Just about everything in our culture fights against moving at a slower pace. Throughout my twenties, I ate all too many meals in front of my computer or while walking around and on the go, stressed out to the max. To be honest, sometimes it still happens because . . . life. But little did I know that my body wouldn't prioritize digesting until I had calmed down and sat down. My body could not process the food I consumed in a hurried/anxious state until I was finally still. That's because when I was rushing around frantically, my body wasn't in the parasympathetic (calm) state needed for optimal digestion.

Anxiety and stress take a large toll on us. They even impair the way we take in nutrients. For instance, we must be calm internally for our digestive systems to properly break down foods and draw out the nutrients. Mindlessly gulping down food once will cause discomfort; when it becomes a regular practice, it will likely contribute to pain, bloating, constipation, and more. The body prioritizes this parasympathetic state so much so that it will literally hold on to the food dumped into your stomach while you're running around and begin to fully digest it once you are able to sit still.

The GI tract is so brilliantly designed that little flaps called sphincters, which are at the top and bottom of the stomach, will remain closed until the stomach and then the small intestine are prepared to digest food. Food and stomach acid in the lower esophagus can lead to heartburn. If food makes it to the stomach but the acidity level is not yet high enough, the food may sit there, leading to digestive symptoms like bloating, gas, and constipation. If the body is under stress, the stomach's role in digestion may take longer than the ideal two to three hours.

The Stomach

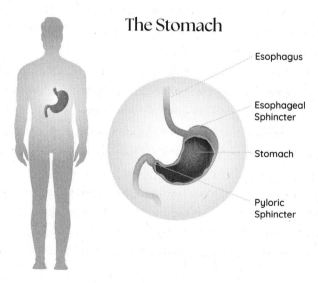

Esophagus

Esophageal
Sphincter

Stomach

Pyloric
Sphincter

A chemical reaction occurs each time stomach acid breaks down food. Enzymes are the proteins in our bodies behind these reactions. Some enzymes are produced by our bodies; we get others through the food we eat. Each type of enzyme has a different assignment; digestive enzymes are produced mainly in the pancreas and small intestine.[1] For example, the digestive enzyme amylase is found in saliva and the pancreas. Its only job is to break down carbohydrates.[2] The more saliva the body produces, the more amylase is available to better break down the carbs we take in. Furthermore, the longer food is in your mouth, the longer amylase has time to work.

The moment you begin thinking about food, your body sends signals to the mouth and stomach to start producing saliva and gastric juice. The longer you give your body the opportunity to really think about the food you're preparing to eat, the more saliva production, the more enzymes, the better breakdown of foods.

This is further evidence of how essential it is to slow down when preparing and consuming food. God designed our bodies in such a strategic way that when we source foods that He provided from the earth and spend time cutting, dicing, smelling, roasting, and seasoning them, our bodies are simultaneously creating the very things they need to break down the foods we are about to eat.

And so our fast-paced way of living—including the abundance of convenience food options—affects our bodies even at the cellular level. When we approach a drive-through window on our way to an appointment and consume food quickly in the car, we are not giving our bodies the signals they need to digest well. A highly processed meal eaten with little thought can inhibit the production of these digestive enzymes in the pancreas, as well as other enzymes elsewhere in the body.

Some signs and symptoms that the body is lacking enzymes

are stomach cramping, stomach pain, gas, nausea, bloating, unexplained weight gain or loss, and weak immune function. Certain foods contain more digestive enzymes than others, and those may be therapeutic. Enzymes like amylase (which breaks down carbs), lipase (which breaks down fats), and protease (which breaks down proteins) can be found in food sources. Here is a partial list:

- avocado
- banana
- kefir
- kiwi
- mango
- papaya
- pineapple
- raw honey
- sauerkraut

Supplementing with digestive enzymes may be necessary in cases of severe digestive issues. If you'd like to explore this option, be sure to consult with a nutritionist or your physician.[3]

Once the gut has received healing through an intentional process such as the Whole-Body Health Protocol, a drive-through here and there is not the end of the world. If you eat this way several times a week, however, your body will be unable to create some of the essential enzymes, causing a deficiency that may trigger digestive issues.

You will benefit whenever you take time to thoughtfully prepare and savor the smells of the food you're about to eat. After that, it's imperative to sit down, eat slowly, and enjoy the meal you've worked so hard on. By being present, you've already prepped your saliva glands to receive food, as well as produced gastric juices to break down the food.

Lingering around the table once a meal is over brings added benefits. Gathering with others after dinner is a lost art, but in ancient times (and in some countries even today) it was a regular practice. I think it was God's intention from the beginning. The body needs us to give it space to complete the digestive process optimally.

SETTING THE TABLE

One way I have learned to promote a parasympathetic state of being for myself and my family is to always keep the table set. Once one meal is finished, I clean the table and immediately set it for the next meal. I also do my best to keep our kitchen cleared, with no piles of mail or clutter on the counters.

When I first started this practice, I wondered whether it was a bit much to bring out full place settings with water and wine glasses, salad plates, and coffee mugs for regular weekday meals. As my husband and I have gotten used to doing this, however, we've found that enjoying even a simple meal of grain-free spaghetti on beautiful plates creates a deep satisfaction and calm as we enjoy the dinner that we've worked hard to prepare and serve.

In addition, when the table is set all day, we are constantly reminded not only to slow down but to worship God as we remember His provision of good food from the beginning of time. It reminds us to invite God into our daily healing space as we walk through the house and prepare dinner at night. Healing isn't linear; it's not a one-and-done type of thing. Yes, we work hard to bring deep healing to the gut, and then we work a different kind of hard—intentional daily practices—to maintain that health.

Parenting little ones can make unhurried time seem like an impossible luxury. Yet as we are able, my husband and I tend to the babies after dinner and then linger as long and as often as we can. Whether at the table, on the couch, or in the study, we might enjoy a piece of extra dark chocolate as we read or catch up with each other after dinner. We've found this intentional practice to be consistently nourishing to our marriage too.

I still remember an evening when our older son, Whitton, was just a month old. Daniel had made a rack of lamb with roasted veggies and potatoes. Rather than hurriedly eating this meal on paper plates on the couch before the baby woke up, my husband plated the food beautifully and we sat at the table with our baby. As I watched Daniel light a candle "just because," I shed some tears because of how intentional and nourishing everything felt. Something about the care taken with that table nourished my soul, healing it just a little more. We ate together very slowly, talked about life as new parents, and really enjoyed our time together. One reason we were able to have this shared experience was because the work of setting the table had already been done. Once the meal was finished and we were ready to eat, all we had to do was light a candle.

Being around a table with friends and family—but with no electronic devices—enables our bodies to enter into a parasympathetic state.

One of my favorite pictures of parasympathetic living is a story in the Old Testament of King David's table, where grace, honor, and unrepayable kindness were displayed.

In David's time, eating with the king at his table was a great honor. A place at this table also meant that the person would be cared for by the king—they were set for life. In 2 Samuel 9, we learn that Mephibosheth, a grandson of the previous king, Saul, had been invited by David to eat at his table. This was significant because Saul and David were enemies. Yet after Saul's death, David didn't shun his predecessor's family or consider them a threat to his throne. Instead, he wanted to show kindness to Mephibosheth, one of Saul's last direct descendants, who had not only been considered an outcast but who was unable to walk due to an injury he suffered as a young boy.

When David first summoned Mephibosheth, Saul's grandson was afraid for his life. Instead of killing him, however, David invited him to dine at his table permanently and restored to him the lands that had once belonged to Saul. Talk about parasympathetic healing. Not only did Mephibosheth no longer need to fear for his life, but he knew he would be generously provided for. This table is such a picture of grace and rest, and it's one reason my husband and I long to create peace at our table and host others as often as we are able.

To be clear, I don't think we have to consume all of our meals in this unhurried state (just as I don't think we have to completely ban sugar from our diet). We are striving for holistic health and healing—not perfection. That's why, just as it's worth asking ourselves what types of food we want to eat the majority of the time, it's valuable to determine how to create an environment where we can regularly eat in a way that will nourish our bodies and souls.

THE ROLE OF SLEEP AND SABBATH

While a nutritious diet is essential for healing the gut and reducing the risk of inflammation and disease, sleep and regular rest play essential roles as well. In chapter 5, we considered how sleep affects our bodies' metabolism, immunity, and hormonal balance. As a reminder, each of our bodies follows a unique circadian rhythm that responds to light and dark and that runs on a twenty-four-hour cycle. This rhythm impacts how we sleep and how well we can focus, process nutrients, regulate blood sugar and hormones, and more.[4] We want the rhythm to follow the sun so that we feel awake during the morning, regulated and energized throughout the day, and then ready to rest when the sun sets. When this rhythm is steady and matches the natural light and darkness, our bodies can appropriately manage hormones and better balance our blood sugar. This is why relying on multiple cups of coffee throughout the day to stay awake and following that with a glass or two of red wine at night to wind down isn't a helpful strategy. This doesn't make coffee or wine "bad"; it just means the body shouldn't need them to wake up or wind down. Our bodies should be capable of doing that on their own.

The Sabbath is another example of a gift God gave that follows a regular rhythm: Once every seven days, we are invited to stop so that we can unplug, rest, and worship. This day of rest is mentioned first in Genesis, and God mentions it again several times after that:

> The heavens and the earth were completed in all their vast array. By the seventh day God had finished the work he had been doing; so on the seventh day he rested from all his work. Then God blessed the seventh day and made it holy, because on it he rested from all the work of creating that he had done.
> GENESIS 2:1-3

> Remember the Sabbath day by keeping it holy.
> EXODUS 20:8

> Observe the Sabbath day by keeping it holy, as the LORD your God has commanded you.
> DEUTERONOMY 5:12

Clearly God did not give the Sabbath to us as an afterthought; instead, it's a command.

The Lord created us to live in and cultivate a mindset of holy rest. That is why He told us to honor Him by observing the Sabbath and stopping to rest. Doing so creates space for deep healing and follows His example of spending six days working to create the world and resting on the seventh. Intentional rest not only allows us to remember Him, but it can help heal our bodies.

Sometimes when we hear the word *command*, we assume we are being asked to do something unpleasant. But while it may be hard to set aside our work one day a week, neglecting to do so is like leaving a lavish gift unopened. Pastor John Mark Comer explains that "the word *Sabbath* comes to us from the Hebrew *Shabbat*. The word literally means 'to stop.' . . . But it can also be translated 'to delight.' It has this dual idea of stopping and also of joying in God."[5]

Comer reminds us that when we do take the time to enjoy this gift, its peaceful effects follow us: "Sabbath is more than just a day; it's a *way of being* in the world. It's a spirit of restfulness that comes from abiding, from living in the Father's loving presence all week long."[6] Resting well doesn't just happen in today's world, however. We have to work hard to rest well.

We cannot fully absorb the goodness of God and receive His blessing with thanksgiving if we do not stop to ponder, wonder, and think on things that are from above. Living at a pace that is unreasonably fast 24-7 never allows us the chance to digest the wonders of the world or to gratefully consider the parts of our lives that are rich in meaning. I've heard someone say that time is a thief, but what if we sometimes stood still and recognized that *we* are in the memories being made that very instant? What if we recognized that we have been the thieves of our own time and can give it back to ourselves? What if we took the time to feel, taste, see, and hear the memories we are making so that when we look back at them, we fully experience how we nourished our souls in times of blessing and times of mourning? What if we deeply processed our times of pain and stress as they were happening by surrendering everything we have and everything we are to a heavenly Father who knows us best and wants to heal our hearts and bodies? We want to fully digest the one life we've been given, and God commands us to pause and remember in order to do so.

Just as the Sabbath is meant for remembering God, it's also intended to be a time dedicated to worshiping Him. This is a full-life posture of orienting our entire selves around Him and who He is. As we do this, we also recenter ourselves as children of God so that we can surrender every part of our day and ourselves to the God who cares more about us than we do.

In the context of food and our relationship with eating and our bodies, the Sabbath is an opportunity to remember that God created the human body for good—to know how to heal itself—and to receive the many blessings of nourishment through real, properly prepared foods. It is a reminder that we can stop our work one day a week, trusting that God will provide everything we need. And in Scripture we see God providing His children with nutritious food and restorative rest time and time again.

THE ROLE OF TRUST IN SABBATH: BREAD FROM HEAVEN

A beautiful illustration of His provision appears in the book of Exodus. God instructs the wandering Israelites, who escaped captivity in Egypt and were on their way to the land God had promised to their forefather Abraham, to gather the food He provided for them every morning. He tells them not to take more than they will need for that day. When it comes to food, it's tempting for you and me to grab more than we need to ensure we'll have enough. The Israelites were no different from us.

The Bible tells us that God provided a substance called manna to meet the nutritional needs of the Israelites while they were in the wilderness, completely dependent on God. "The people of Israel called the bread manna. It was white like coriander seed and tasted like wafers made with honey" (Exodus 16:31). Manna was God's divine rescue plan, and it sustained the Israelites for forty years in the wilderness.

We've talked a lot in this book about the importance of eating real foods, so you may be curious about what coriander seed is, where it comes from, and its nutritional benefits.

Coriander, also known as cilantro, is native to Asia and southern Europe, though it now grows in many parts of the world. Though many people like to use cilantro leaves in cooking, the coriander seeds are delicious themselves. Not only that, but they are full of nutritional benefits. Among other things, they

are rich in copper, zinc, iron, and other essential minerals
     that the body needs for every enzymatic activity,
help to increase metabolism,
help fuel the thyroid for proper function,
are packed with nutrients and various anti-inflammatory
     antioxidants,
help stabilize blood sugar, and
promote healthy digestion and good gut health.[7]

This list includes just about everything a human needs to function optimally. Although many biblical scholars believe manna resembled, rather than tasted like, coriander seed,[8] I am struck by the nutritional richness of both. God *knew* what His people needed to make it through the treacherous wilderness, and He packed those nutrients into this bread-like wafer.

Interestingly, new manna appeared every morning—except on the Sabbath. Six days a week any manna remaining on the ground melted later that day, while any manna the Israelites tried to hoard became full of maggots. On the seventh day, the Sabbath, however, God still prioritized rest and worship. So He told the people that, on the day before the Sabbath, they should gather enough manna to last two days: "This is what the LORD commanded: 'Tomorrow is to be a day of sabbath rest, a holy sabbath to the LORD. So bake what you want to bake and boil what you want to boil. Save whatever is left and keep it until morning'" (Exodus 16:23). Once again, some Israelites revealed their doubt by trying to find manna on the Sabbath, only to endure the Lord's rebuke: "'How long will you refuse to keep my commands and my instructions? Bear in mind that the LORD has given you the Sabbath; that is why on the sixth day he gives you bread for two days. Everyone is to stay where they are on the seventh day; no one is to go out.' So the people rested on the seventh day" (verses 28-30). Clearly, God wanted His people to trust Him to supply every need of their bodies and souls—particularly nutritious food, adequate rest, and His faithful love. Even today, observing the Sabbath enables us to remember and rejoice.

Upon entering the Promised Land—a region "flowing with milk and honey" (Exodus 3:8)—the Israelites were given an abundance of delicious foods. Because they understood God's provision after the season of "drought and fasting" in the wilderness, when they had to rely completely on Him for nourishment and rest, they didn't need to go crazy on the other side. They didn't have to overindulge because they knew, by God's grace, that they would never have to go without again. They could indulge freely and worshipfully, and the Sabbath was a regular opportunity to remember God's mercy and goodness together.

In the New Testament, recalling this divine rescue, Jesus identifies himself with manna. Jesus is the true Bread of Life that comes down from heaven (see John 6:32). When people are most vulnerable to themselves and to life on earth—hungry for more than what this life has to offer—God longs to nourish humans with salvation from Himself. He longs to be the Bread of Life, the bread of nourishment for the longing soul. He also promises to bring us rest (see Matthew 11:28). Manna from heaven is a divine exchange. It's God stepping into humanity and humans preparing for eternal life with Him.

Today when we honor and remember the Sabbath, we can pause, stop, and take delight. As we slow down, we can enjoy our food with gratitude and thankfulness. We don't have to obsess over what we are putting in our bodies and mull over what it's doing to us physically. We trust that God gave us bodies that know how to heal themselves as we partake of delicious, real food.

Because Sabbath is an act of worship, how can you incorporate food into this time of quiet celebration? What feels worshipful? Long meals with friends? Dinner on the patio with your partner or kids? Enjoying a plated dinner by yourself? Think on whatever draws you to consider the magnitude of God's goodness and make it your way of worshipful eating. You don't have to do this at every meal, but a lifestyle of worshipful eating allows you the space to be more attuned to the greatness of God and His provision rather than worrying about and/or being paralyzed by what food might be doing to your body.

Remembering God and resting in His presence also enable us to process any shame we have around food as we allow God to replace those feelings with nourishment from the inside out.

And as we make food preparation and mealtimes priorities in our days, our focus moves from seeing food as either a necessary evil or something to soothe ourselves in secret to viewing it as a way to enjoy God's gifts with those closest to us.

Tips for Resting and De-stressing

1. Engage in quiet activities like journaling, walking, and listening to spa music while resting at home. Avoid scrolling through your phone as you do so.
2. Spend some time with God each day, even if it's as simple as remembering that He is with you as you sit quietly.
3. Read a book just for fun.
4. Create a bedtime routine that helps prepare your body to relax. Sprinkle a few drops of lavender or peppermint oil on your pillowcase and take some deep breaths before falling asleep. This will promote the production of melatonin while reducing cortisol creation.
5. Get a new set of place mats for your dinner table and freshen it with flowers. Try resetting the table after you finish each meal so you can slow down and enjoy the next one.

digging deeper

1. What is your typical posture when eating? Do you tend to eat in the car or standing up, or do you typically take the time to sit down and enjoy your food? What might you do differently going forward?
2. What keeps you from eating mindfully? What is one practice you could try this week to eat in a more restful way?

3. How would you rate the quality of your sleep? What is one habit you could try this week to sleep better at night?

4. How might unwanted stress/trauma be preventing you from getting the rest and nourishment your body needs, whether through food, sleep, or the Sabbath?

5. In what ways do you practice the Sabbath weekly or rest daily?

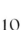

10

FEAST OF HIS FAITHFULNESS

EATING WITH DELIGHT WHEN FOOD
BECOMES ENJOYABLE AGAIN

When I hear the word *feast*, I immediately think of one of the first Easters I celebrated in Texas. I gathered with several friends for a dinner hosted by a family from our church. Once I arrived at their home, I was greeted and invited to find my place around their table, indicated by a personalized nameplate and a bottle of my favorite beverage. Within thirty seconds of entering a house full of people ready to feast, I felt seen, known, and loved. Any tremor of discomfort I'd felt at celebrating this holiday in a brand-new city instantly dissipated.

The table was set with colorful plates and yellow linen napkins artfully folded in silver napkin rings. Silver serving dishes were piled high with raw cheese, honey, and nuts. Everything went together beautifully. Once we had all gathered, the lamb and roasted veggies were brought out as well. Somehow because of the profound pleasure I got from the nourishing foods in front of us, I deeply sensed Christ's resurrection. It was the first time I remember being fully present with those around me, taking in every second as a holy moment of celebration. Good food has a way of reaching deep inside us to touch the exact parts of our souls that need to be awakened.

We sat around the table for hours, remembering God's goodness and sharing stories. By now, I had been working with a therapist and nutritionist for quite a while, so when I was served nourishing foods that tasted so delicious, I no longer felt as if I were "cheating"; my body and mind could relax and enjoy them while remaining present to everyone around me. I didn't regret a single thing I ate, and I remember just about everything—even the coffee, iconic Texas pecan. As that was served, I noticed that each of the guests had the same kind of coffee mug—just in different colors. Through laughter, tears, and storytelling, everyone gripped their mugs a little tighter and leaned in a little bit closer as conversation flowed. It was meaningful and soothing. For the first time in a decade, I didn't lament the food I was consuming, beat myself up for eating something sweet, or long for more self-control.

As if the dinner experience alone weren't enough to heal just a little bit more of my soul, as we ended the night we were told to take our coffee mugs with us. Our host explained that they had been hand-selected for us as a way to remember this night with nourishing foods and good friends. Daniel and I have since adopted this small but powerful gesture of giving guests a personalized coffee mug when hosting family and friends on special occasions.

I am a foodie, and deep down have always been, so getting to enjoy delicious foods during a meaningful celebration makes me want to skip and dance. This Easter feast was the first time I fully realized this about myself and embraced it. If you've had any kind of negative history with food, especially overeating, the concept of feasting might produce feelings of guilt. I get it. My prayer is that this chapter brings freedom rather than fear or restriction. Freedom around the table doesn't mean loading up on anything you want but rather gathering with others and intentionally preparing, serving, and enjoying foods that are both indulgent and nourishing.

FEASTING NOW AND THEN

Did you know that feasting is a recurrent theme in the Bible? Pastor, author, and biblical scholar John Piper defines feasting as "the enjoyment of abundance" and a time of remembrance. Several different feasts and festivals are mentioned in the Old Testament, including the feasts of Passover, the First Fruits, Trumpets, and Pentecost. Each one of them, established by God Himself, was an invitation to the Israelites to celebrate with one another as they enjoyed God's abundant gifts and remembered His goodness and mercy.[1]

Scripture frequently speaks of feasting as a gift from God:

On this mountain the LORD Almighty will prepare
    a feast of rich food for all peoples,
a banquet of aged wine—
    the best of meats and the finest of wines.
On this mountain he will destroy
    the shroud that enfolds all peoples,
the sheet that covers all nations;

> he will swallow up death forever.
> The Sovereign LORD will wipe away the tears
> from all faces;
> he will remove his people's disgrace
> from all the earth.
> The LORD has spoken.

ISAIAH 25:6-8

How appealing does it sound to sit at the top of a mountain with the Lord to enjoy a feast of rich food, including "the best of meats," and fine wine to celebrate our redemption? This passage speaks of the feast we will enjoy when Christ returns. It also reflects His loving provision for the Israelites. After they wandered for years in the wilderness, often hopeless and struggling, the Lord brought them out and settled them in the Promised Land, where they were allowed to feast. Best of all, God offered Himself, removing their tears and disgrace.

The psalmist also rejoiced in the generous character of God, specifically mentioning feasting as one expression of that:

> Your righteousness is like the highest mountains,
> your justice like the great deep.
> You, LORD, preserve both people and animals.
> How priceless is your unfailing love, O God!
> People take refuge in the shadow of your wings.
> They feast on the abundance of your house;
> you give them drink from your river of delights.
> For with you is the fountain of life;
> in your light we see light.

PSALM 36:6-9

Feasting is *meant* to be a shared experience. Having said that, when I was single, feasting with others was a rare occurrence. But once I began to eat real foods with gratitude in my heart, mealtime became a time of joyful contentment anyway. Still, the temptation to overindulge decreases when feasting with others because the focus is not solely on the food but on bringing people around a table to enjoy and mark sacred moments. Food enhances the experience of the celebratory communion with those you love. Feasting alone doesn't have the same impact. Quite frankly, the feasting foods never taste as good when you indulge by yourself.

Of course, we live in the twenty-first century, and food and preparation methods are much different now than they were in biblical times. Because food is so readily available—particularly processed foods—we could "feast" at just about every meal if we wanted. The feasts we read about in the Bible are much different. Regularly indulging in sweets and packaged snacks is not what God had in mind when celebrating the feasts of His people.

Thankfully God knew the challenges we would face today and offers us grace in all things. While I don't think we should be legalistic about what we eat, nor am I saying that we can never eat another chocolate chip cookie, I do believe we need to be aware of the posture of our hearts and strive to consume food as God intended whenever possible. We are up against so many challenges in today's fast-paced world, but we can still eat real foods designed to bring us health and healing.

Food is absolutely a form of holy nourishment. Yes, it fuels our bodies, but it also fuels the way we participate in life on this earth. It directly impacts how we view God, relate to God, and love God. It directly impacts how we love ourselves and others, and how we show up for the assignments God gives us on this earth. How we choose to nourish our bodies is a direct yes or no to showing up for this one beautiful life God has given us to live.

Once you begin to look at food as a holy nourishment, preparing and consuming it with intention, your body will begin to heal, your urges will be tamed, and your entire self—body and soul—will be nourished. Feasting well will become something you want to create time for, even if it means staying up late, getting up early, or washing a few more dishes. In addition, the desire and urge to reach for packaged and processed food will diminish.

When I began studying nutrition and working on my own health years ago, I didn't yet realize that the Lord took pleasure in my enjoyment of His good gifts, namely real, nourishing foods, especially in the company of others. What a delight to recognize that feasting was designed by God as a way for His people to enjoy life and worship Him!

FIXING TO FEAST

We cannot feast well if we are focused only on food. Feasting is about the entire experience of remembering God's provision and grace. As you begin to see food as God's good gift, meant to be savored and enjoyed with others, now is the time to take control of your life and your relationship with food. The most important thing you can do at the outset is to reach deep within your soul, invite God in, and determine *why* you want to heal your gut and change your lifestyle for good. What pain points might be stopping you from living your life to the absolute fullest? How might you begin to tend to those? I pray for you now, friend, that you will have the courage to ask God to step into those hidden areas of your soul with His grace. He cares about where you've been, what you've done, and what's happened to you.

I can't tell you that even the most natural, nutrient-rich food will make your life perfect, take away any kind of pain, or be the answer to everything in an instant. You don't need a quick fix or another person to tell you to claw your way out or to just "be okay." What I can tell you is that real food given by God is designed to nourish and enhance the healing process in your mind, body, and soul. You're fine just where you are, and God isn't afraid of your pain, your past, your story, or your desires for the future. But when you're ready, God will meet you where you are. He won't leave you there, though; He will take you somewhere better. I pray that in that moment you will have the perseverance to lean into a healing protocol and trust that while you do deep work, God will do something even deeper in your heart and soul on a divine and cellular level because He loves you.

Despite the inevitable ups and downs, eating real food and limiting sugar is the direction you want to be heading. Having a gut that is strong and able to function properly is what makes the moments of feasting so impactful. While you can partake in a feast on celebratory occasions even if you're still striving to improve your eating habits, there is so much more freedom on the other side of healing.

As we move toward the end of the book, I want to leave you with some final ideas I offer my clients as we work toward whole-body healing.

Aim for consistency, not perfection

For optimal physical, spiritual, and emotional health, I estimate that you should eat nutritious foods in moderation 80 to 90 percent of the time. The body is resilient and can then handle a 10 to 20 percent range of feasting. Food touches taste receptors in our mouths and pleasure centers in our brains that I believe God intended to be touched. As you shift from mindless to mindful eating, you can trust that your body was created by God to know how to heal itself and that He wants a life of abundance for you just as much as you do.

When you eat in moderation, you are not forcing yourself to eat nothing or to eat bland foods. You are simply rejecting the addictions of sugar, gluten, and stress that bring havoc to your system. You are saying no to inflammatory foods in order to say yes to the foods that nourish your body. This may be hard at first, but during the transition to proper nourishment, you are trading your selfish addictions for something greater—the health and energy that will allow you to show up for yourself, your family, and your calling to the absolute fullest.

Look upward, not inward, for self-control

Are you controlled by the narrative that you do not have self-control and never will? Let today be the day that you fully and completely let that go. When you begin addressing disordered eating patterns and emotional pain at their root, you'll learn that you have a lot more strength and resiliency than you ever thought possible. That's because God is just waiting for you to invite Him into your commitment to health: "The fruit of the Spirit is love, joy, peace, patience, kindness, goodness, faithfulness, gentleness, self-control; against such things there is no law. And those who belong to Christ Jesus have crucified the flesh with its passions and desires" (Galatians 5:22-24, ESV).

When self-control becomes a divine surrender rather than a fleshly desire, there is an exchange of self for something far greater than you could ever comprehend. Yes, lifestyle changes may seem beneficial, even gratifying, in the moment. But when you exchange, by faith, that longing for instant gratification for a commitment to making lasting change, you pave a path for God to do something even greater.

It's important to keep reminding yourself of the "why" behind your decision to change the way you source, prepare, and choose foods. That way, when motivation fails you, your desire for renewed health will sustain you. Here are a few mindset shifts that may help:

- Make a decision before you have to make a decision.
- Choose to start and choose not to stop.
- Don't rely on your feelings to carry you through the entire journey.

With such a mindset, temptation will begin to fall away. Yes, it's hard at times, and the Whole-Body Health Protocol is not magic. It can take a while to unlearn bad habits and relearn how to properly fuel your body, but once you've grasped how to do it and have really determined why you want to nourish and heal your body, temptation will become less of a battle. Eating foods that are not good for you slowly becomes a nonissue when you fully understand and grasp God's assignment for your life while you're on earth. You cannot function optimally and properly if you're not nourishing your body from dust to dust. It's that simple.

The eighteenth-century preacher and author John Wesley followed a strict daily regimen to remain physically and spiritually healthy. Interestingly, it appears that Wesley followed the regimen as a means to gain self-control; he didn't see it as evidence that he had already mastered it. He described such habits as following a healthy diet and waking early as means God used to help him grow in the fruit of the Spirit. In other words, he saw "a daily health regimen [as] a cooperative endeavour between humans and God."[2]

We will always be faced with challenges when it comes to pursuing a lifestyle of holy nourishment. These challenges will look different for each of us, but God can work even through our difficulties and failures: "No discipline seems pleasant at the time, but painful. Later on, however, it produces a harvest of righteousness and peace for those who have been trained by it" (Hebrews 12:11).

Value variety

Eating healthy doesn't have to look like baking a batch of chicken breasts without flavoring that you then pair with sides of broccoli and sweet potatoes for seven days in a row. In fact, your gut can't handle the same kind of food over and over again. It needs a variety of nutrients to produce good bacteria, maintain a balanced microbiome, and keep your immune system strong.[3]

Ever heard the phrase "eat the rainbow"? This is something to take to heart. It's not so much about overthinking the exact nutritional makeup of each food as it is focusing on eating a variety of real foods. Don't be afraid to try new foods, cook new meats, and sauté or roast new veggies.

Invite a friend or loved one to plan and prep with you

Fighting against the modern food industry and figuring out how to avoid synthetic ingredients and processed items can be hard sometimes—especially when you're trying to do it on your own. Have you ever had a day when you first thought about dinner plans at five o'clock as you were walking in the front door after a long car pool or day of meetings? To reduce stress and avoid the temptation to just order a pizza, I suggest that you plan and prep for your meals once a week—preferably with someone else.

You could work alongside your spouse or roommate if they are on board with the changes you are making. If you live by yourself, you might call up a friend to join you on weekends, alternating between homes where you can cook, meal prep, and plan, making the experience just as enjoyable as the eating. When I was single, a friend and I met for meal planning and prep once a week. We shopped together, splitting the bill 50/50, and then meal prepped every Sunday.

You can make meal prep a nourishing event in itself. Get out your favorite glass, pour your favorite beverage, and turn on some calming music. You might use this time to pray over your body and the nourishment it will receive that week. Whether you're working to heal your body or you've moved on to making lasting lifestyle changes, allow God to be a part of everything—even your advance preparations.

Having someone in your corner—be it a spouse, roommate, friend, or family member—makes this kind of food lifestyle easier, more enjoyable, and more profound.

Limit sweets—especially when you're alone

While avoiding sugar whenever possible is advisable, it's especially important to limit indulging in sweet foods when you're alone—particularly if you struggle with sugar addiction, emotional eating, or a lack of control. Eating indulgent foods alone often leads to negative thoughts about your emotions, self-control, and even your body. The temptation to beat yourself up will almost always be greater after you've eaten a pint of ice cream in the living room by yourself than when you've enjoyed a scoop while out with friends. If you use indulgent foods as a way to soothe difficult feelings or to cope with a bad day or a tough situation, you may be trying to self-medicate using comfort foods. In the end, it will be far more satisfying to process those feelings with a safe person.

On the other hand, the ice cream served with the wedding cake at your best friend's wedding should be enjoyed! Rather than hearing a tiny voice inside saying, *You shouldn't be eating that*, eating the food should actually be *fun*. It is likely served on a pretty dish, and you enjoy it while focusing on the people around you. The pleasure center in your brain magnifies the celebration at hand. You might even notice how delicious it tastes because you can enjoy the flavors while you eat it. If only real ingredients were used to make that ice cream, even better. Your body recognizes it as something to break down, process, and use for good. In this setting, the temptation to overindulge has been drastically reduced, and both your tongue and your soul are touched with a holy satisfaction of real nourishment as you celebrate with those you love.

Does this mean that when you're surrounded by people, it's okay to indulge? I cannot tell you how many clients I've seen over the years who have been riddled with guilt over office snacks. Here's what I recommend: Prepare nourishing meals and snacks that you can take to work and skip the treats in your break room. It doesn't matter if your coworkers look at you funny or if someone begs you to partake. When I was in this situation, at first my coworkers were confused and tried to tempt me to snack when I didn't grab a donut or cookie. But after a few weeks they applauded me for my discipline and eventually asked me how I was able to withstand temptation because they wanted that too.

Linger longer when you can

I've already told you about the third date with my husband, Daniel—the carefully prepared meal he made when I knew I was in love with him! In all seriousness, he made this meal over five years ago, and I still remember it because of the intentionality and detail that went into it. We lingered for hours over that special meal and a good bottle of red wine. That is what simple feasting looked like for us on a random Wednesday. We were celebrating and learning about each other, swapping stories, and remembering God's goodness. Neither of us worried that anything on the table was something we "shouldn't eat" or might eat "too much" of. When food is real and nourishing, it's deeply satisfying.

Of course, the fact that it was one very special and significant event is the reason I remember that dinner so well. But it was just the first of many times when we've intentionally lingered a little bit longer at our dinner table. Doing so gives our bodies a chance to digest calmly as intended and our minds and souls a chance to settle after a busy day. Now it's also a chance for Daniel and me to model calmness and connect with our two little ones.

Take control when you eat out

I was single for several years after moving to Houston. One blind date changed all that. For our first meeting, I dressed up to meet Daniel at an upscale restaurant with many healthy but interesting food options. I had been somewhat nervous when he suggested we meet at a restaurant because I knew that eating out could be a challenge—not impossible, but a challenge. I didn't say anything beforehand because I didn't want to be "that person."

I was surprised when he ordered in a similar way to how I order when eating out. He asked for salmon but requested they hold the butter sauce. Though that dish was typically served with buttery garlic mashed potatoes and a fried vegetable curry, he requested a big salad with no croutons instead. He shamelessly and quietly modified the meal as it appeared on the menu to comply with the way he had chosen to nourish his body. Daniel and I have debriefed this first date many times because I think his "no-fuss" adjustments were a prelude to me falling hard for him. In fact, I've learned from him that real foods are actually tastier than anything processed when you slow down to pair flavors and take time to cook.

So what does this mean for you? First, recognize that eating out can get complicated, but there are some steps you can take to modify dishes to make them healthier. In general it's best to ask for items that are baked or steamed. Many restaurants use soybean oil, so I recommend requesting that an alternative cooking oil, like olive or avocado, be used if possible.

NO BETTER TIME THAN NOW

If you recognize that you generally eat alone and that your diet centers around processed foods, there is hope. It begins by working on bringing healing and alignment to the gut, perhaps even being intentional about removing trigger foods.

Not every meal needs to be gourmet—in fact, most of them will not be. It's possible to detach from feelings of deprivation when you consider all the good you're doing for your body, mind, and spirit. Remember, too, that God is a gracious and generous Father who intends to supply all of your needs, including nutritious food.

Most of us, especially in America, are not deprived of food so we must *choose* to eat in moderation. What does that look like? I am speaking of the choice to "under" indulge—choosing not to eat every food available to us exactly when we want it. Because we have access to numerous grocery stores and fast-food outlets, food is everywhere. We typically don't have physical pangs of hunger to remind us of how reliant we must be on the Spirit to feed us; as a result, it's very easy to submit to every craving and completely miss the deeper blessing God wants to offer to satisfy our longings—Himself.

Jesus shows us how we can rely on God and His Word to overcome temptation around food. When He was tempted by Satan himself during an extremely vulnerable time, Jesus responded by immediately surrendering to His Father. Right after His baptism, Jesus was led into the wilderness where He fasted for forty days and nights. He was then tempted by the devil to turn stones into bread. Of course, Jesus was hungry, but rather than giving in to the tempter, He said, "Man shall not live on bread alone, but on every word that comes from the mouth of God" (Matthew 4:4). In that moment, His need for physical nourishment was transformed, and God the Father supernaturally supplied Him with every need as a result of His obedience.

Feasting is wonderful in the right context, but "famine" can be as well. You must lean on the Lord for His power and provision. In these times of growing dependence, deep change happens as you move toward a holy desire to want what God wants for your body. By rejecting some modern conveniences and processed foods, you're giving God room to give you Himself. As you quiet the distractions and learn how to nourish yourself, you're accepting the abundant life God offers to you by His grace. So often we think we have to be self-reliant, but I think it's just the opposite. Only through dependence on God can we learn to control and discipline our desires for God's glory. (Please note that this paragraph on famine is intended for those who struggle with overindulging or avoiding certain foods at times. If you struggle instead with severely limiting or working off your food intake, I advise that you seek wise counsel from a Christian counselor, nutrition practitioner, or both so you can learn to enjoy adequate amounts of real food without guilt.)

Avoiding office snacks or the fantastic grocery story deal on frozen pizza is not a deprivation once eating becomes a daily act of worship. Foods that are not nourishing to your body are not even remotely nourishing to your soul. You are invited to something greater.

Saying no means saying yes to internal neurotransmitters and messengers sending appropriate signals throughout the body to work for you and not against you. Saying no means that you get to show up for the *one* life God has gifted you with. When eating becomes something holy, saying no isn't about your waistline or your blood pressure or your willpower; it's about inviting God to direct one of the most impactful tools you have while living on earth—your health and wellness.

The shift doesn't always happen overnight, and for some people it's not that simple. I get it. There are a lot of layers when it comes to food, healing, and lifestyle changes. It's an emotional, physical, spiritual, and mental process. Start where you are and offer yourself tender grace when you think you've slipped up. Think how different it would be if the only food available to you was real food, none of which was off-limits? Does that sound scary? That's okay. It may feel intimidating, and it may feel liberating. Either way, this kind of freedom is within closer reach than you think.

You aren't striving for a perfect life or perfect stress-free meals 24-7; you are striving to seek God in every moment, in every nutrient, in every stage of healing for as long as you are here on earth. It looks different for everyone; it can even look different for each of us on different days and in transforming seasons. This particular healing journey is about you and God and anyone you choose to be a part of it.

Invite God to be in on this journey with you! Don't fall for the lie that He's mad at you or ashamed of you for longing for something greater. Instead, believe that if Jesus didn't live on bread alone, then you don't need to either. That means fostering a deep dependency on Him in every area of your life, including your health, no matter what stage you are in or where you are headed.

Here's to no more office party woes. No more struggle around "good" and "bad" foods. No more fad diets that include synthetic foods and shakes. No more shame around where you've been or where you've come from. Here's to relishing the good gifts of the real rainbow of foods and your remarkable body. You, my friend, are gorgeous in every way!

Tips for Feasting Well

1. Consider working with a nutrition practitioner, mental health counselor, or both to begin addressing addictions to any food or food group.
2. When planning and prepping meals, use ingredients that are as close to the source as possible.
3. When you are not in control of the food or meal, enjoy as much as you can from real ingredients. When enjoying a celebratory or milestone event, recognize that some indulgence may be worth it. Once you've laid a good foundation, indulging here and there will not ruin your progress or set you back.
4. Find ways to engage in meaningful conversation and activities whenever you gather to feast with loved ones, whether to celebrate a special occasion or just enjoy being together!

digging deeper

1. If you are tempted to "feast" on sweet treats when you are alone, what is one step you can take to kick that habit to the curb?

2. How can you focus on feasting well when you are celebrating with others? If you find yourself consumed by what's on your plate, how might identifying the root sources of your discomfort help? How can you let go of those negative feelings?

3. After a special occasion, how can you ensure that you can easily move back into your regular routine?

4. How might you invite God into your times of feasting? How do you think that would affect your experience?

APPENDIX A

Whole-Body Health Protocol

This 75-day nutrition plan is designed to be a crucial starting point on your healing journey.* As we've seen, whatever health challenge you face can likely be traced back to the gut. Yes, diet, lifestyle, and supplement routines may vary from person to person; however, lasting transformation generally begins once your GI tract is healthy. This plan calls for strict changes up front to relieve your body of stress caused by food or your environment, giving it the space it needs to heal. Although the program may seem challenging at first, it is meant to give you freedom, not to restrict you.

As you'll see, the first thirty days focus on opening up any compromised detoxification or drainage pathways *before* you begin the six-week Whole-Body Health Protocol, when you'll work to balance the gut microbiome through diet, lifestyle, and (optional) supplements. The body is resilient, and some people see great improvement in as little as two weeks, but for others it takes longer. People in my practice generally need an average of six weeks to see improvement and make lasting changes. Some bodies might

---

* Please note: The recommendations in this protocol are generally safe for most people in good health. If you have any underlying medical issue, are pregnant or nursing, or are on any medications, it is essential that you consult with your health-care provider prior to starting this protocol.

need even more than these two and a half months, so I've designed the protocol to be supportive to the body for up to six months.

No matter how quickly you see results, the Whole-Body Health Protocol will not only help you feel better now but also establish healthy habits to last a lifetime. After all, it takes an *average* of 66 days to establish habits that will be harder to break.[1]

Once your symptoms have resolved or you stop noticing improvements, you'll know that it's time to transition into a more sustainable lifestyle. If you plan to remain on any of the recommended supplements for longer than five to six months, it is best to reach out to a practitioner for help. I also recommend contacting a health practitioner in your area at that point if you're still having issues. If you have experienced chronic pain for months or years, you might also benefit from getting your gut tested. Many nutritionists can complete a GI-MAP evaluation, which reveals the kind and amount of bacteria—both good and bad—in your gut.

Unless your diet already consists of mostly whole foods, you won't want to return to your "normal" way of eating after the protocol ends. Instead, you'll want to transition into a more gut-healthy way of living so that you continue to stay on a path of healing in your body.

This plan does not come with a guarantee from me that you will be healed in six weeks. I'm not promising to solve all your food-related problems, and I definitely do not want you to view this as another "trendy diet." However, this plan is designed to help you pay attention to what you're putting into your body and make some significant changes. It has improved hundreds of lives already; in fact, I led a group of about three hundred people through this plan several years ago, and the feedback was overwhelmingly positive. Nonetheless, there is not a one-size-fits-all plan for life because we are all made so uniquely and wonderfully different. That's why I work one-on-one with clients to get deeper into the root of personal struggles.

With that said, I know enough about the human body and the way God created us to know that this plan serves as an incredible tool for almost everyone because it can initiate deep healing of the gut at root level. The first step toward healing (and for some, the only step) will be to do a massive overhaul or reset, which is what this plan provides.

BREAKING IT ALL DOWN AT THE ROOT—FOR THE RESET

This reset is intended to strengthen your digestive system by increasing good bacteria and removing stressors that contribute to opportunistic bacterial overgrowth and inflammation. The plan features foods and supplements that are specifically designed to bring deep healing. If you've experienced digestive difficulties, abdominal bloating and/or pain, hormone issues, an inability to lose weight, chronic skin issues, or extreme amounts of stress, resetting your digestive system can be the key that unlocks the door to healing in each of these areas.

This plan is different from a fad diet because it's not a one-and-done protocol that you follow only until you have permission to go back to mindless eating. Instead, you'll want to make a mental shift, deciding that you want this to be a new way of life for you.

This is an overview of the plan you'll follow for the next two and a half months:

1. Clear drainage pathways

When entering into a strategic detox, you'll want to be sure that toxins and waste products have a way out of your system. If you usually have one or two bowel movements a day, that's a sign that your body is doing its job to remove waste. As you begin addressing gut imbalances, you want the bad bacteria to have an exit route out of the body rather than recirculate in your intestines, organs, and blood. This will ensure that the rest of the protocol is as effective as possible.

2. Follow a healthy diet

Build your diet on whole and unprocessed foods that are free of synthetic chemicals. (For a refresher on all the characteristics of real foods, see pages 15–16.) Appendix C includes a comprehensive list of foods to enjoy and foods to avoid, but in general, the following points encapsulate what to look for when planning your meals and snacks:

- Consume whole foods, including animal meats and fats, whole fruits and veggies, sprouted or soaked nuts and grains, and anti-inflammatory seeds.
- Avoid refined sugars, gluten, dairy, and soy.
- When shopping for food, avoid items in the center of the grocery store as much as possible, with the exception of organic condiments and herbs and spices.
- Avoid over-the-counter medications and NSAIDs like Advil and Aleve (with your doctor's approval). These medications are helpful in certain situations, but they also are likely to stress the digestive system and can contribute to unwanted bacterial overgrowth.

3. Consider adding gut-healing supplements

I have found that supplements always enhance this process, but you don't necessarily need them all. (See appendix D for a comprehensive list of those that I have found to be most helpful for digestive-related issues.) When it comes to supplements and herbs, there is no one formula for everyone to follow. Because people respond differently to various products, I've included a variety of options.

When selecting supplements, look for products whose quality has been verified by third-party testing, which is indicated by seals on the packaging from NSF International, US Pharmacopeia, UL Solutions, and/or ConsumerLab. Also, if you're pregnant, nursing, or on other medications, or if you're being treated for other health conditions, you'll want to consult with your health-care provider before taking supplements or herbs. (Note: I advise that you take herbs only under the guidance of your practitioner or while you're on the healing protocol, not long term.)

4. When appropriate, address specific digestive issues

Many diseases begin in the gut, and healing can begin there as well. In order for your body to properly absorb nutrients and eliminate toxins, a healthy digestive system is critical. Every cell and chemical messenger, including the neurotransmitters from the brain to the gut, depend on the digestive system to provide nutrients so they can function well. It's important for the GI tract to function properly so your body can handle a gut-healing protocol. That's why, in addition to recommending that you consume real foods and supplements for improved gut health, I suggest that you use some of the herbs recommended on the following page if you suffer from acid reflux/gastroesophageal reflux disease (GERD). (If your symptoms are chronic or have been getting worse, be sure to check with your doctor before trying to address them on your own.)

It's best to be symptom-free of reflux for fourteen to twenty-one days prior to beginning the Whole-Body Health Protocol. Remember that some of the most common symptoms of

GERD—such as heartburn or difficulty swallowing—are not normal. If you've come to rely on acid blockers and/or proton pump inhibitors, it will be important to seek out a practitioner in your area who can help you reverse this. As we've learned, any supplement that blocks acid production will exacerbate the problem by reducing stomach acid. With that being said, you might try one of these supplements (following the dosage instructions on the label and talking with your doctor about potential interactions with other medications) if you suffer from acid reflux:

- Deglycyrrhizinated licorice (DGL)—While having this supplement on hand to soothe the symptoms of heartburn is helpful, you should not rely on it alone. If the discomfort becomes chronic, you'll want to address the deeper issue by working with a practitioner in your area.

- The following herbs generally support healing and soothe the upper GI tract:
  - aloe vera
  - L-glutamine
  - marshmallow root
  - slippery elm
  - vitamin U

DAYS 1–30:

Support body's natural detoxification channels

Irregular or infrequent bowel movements may be an indication that your body is unable to remove waste and toxins effectively. Other signs of compromised drainage pathways include

- chronic inflammation
- chronic infections
- chronic stress
- inability to lose weight
- psoriasis
- eczema
- high cholesterol
- hormone imbalance
- mood swings
- extreme fatigue
- brain fog
- morning stiffness

- parasites
- candida
- swollen glands
- varicose veins
- cellulite
- inability to sweat (or takes a long time)
- bad body smells
- kidney problems
- difficulty recovering from sickness

If constipation is a frequent issue for you, you might extend this first phase of the protocol by another month to offer additional support to the detoxification pathways. As an alternative, you might work one-on-one with a functional practitioner to address any underlying issues.

1. SUPPORT DIGESTION

Here are some supplements and herbs that can promote good digestion. As a general rule, the first thirty-day phase of the program begins here:

Choose one or two digestive supplements to take with each meal. Choose any combination or tinctures that combine a few of these herbs.

In my clinical experience, I've found there is not a one-size-fits-all combination. All of the following supplements and herbs mentioned can be helpful, but it's not necessary to use each of them. As a starting place, I've noted some of the top areas of digestive health each of these potentially supports. Remember that it's important to (1) talk with your doctor to ensure the supplements you choose can be safely taken with your medications and (2) follow the dosage instructions on product labels.

Supplements

- apple cider vinegar—boosts metabolism, helps break down foods
- berberine—balances blood sugar and acts as an antimicrobial
- bromelain—relieves pain in the stomach
- digestive enzymes—help the body break down foods
- betaine hydrochloric acid (HCl) with pepsin—helps supplement stomach acid when your body is depleted
- magnesium—relieves constipation
- whole foods fiber—promotes healthy, daily bowel movements

Herbs

You can take these in isolation; tinctures with these ingredients are also available.

- aloe vera—relieves constipation and stomach pain
- black cumin—serves as an antifungal and helps relieve constipation
- black walnut—expels parasites
- chamomile—relieves upset stomach/indigestion
- clove—serves as an antibacterial (Note: Because this is an antibacterial, take it at a different time of day than a probiotic. It will kill some of the good bacteria while also

cleaning up yeast overgrowth. If used topically, apply just a drop or two of the liquid directly on the throat, once a day.)

- dandelion—supports detoxification of the liver and aids in digestion
- digestive bitters—help the body break down foods
- fennel—addresses constipation
- garlic—boosts immunity and serves as an antifungal
- oregano oil—serves as an antibacterial and targets yeast buildup (Note: Because this oil is an antibacterial, take it at a different time of day than a probiotic. It will kill some of the good bacteria while also cleaning up yeast overgrowth. If used topically, apply just a drop or two of the liquid directly on the throat, once a day.)
- Spanish black radish—helps detoxify the liver and cleanse the colon

Lifestyle habits
- Chew food slowly and up to thirty times per bite.
- Eat while sitting down.
- Eat in a relaxed state as much as possible.

2. BALANCE BLOOD SUGAR

It's essential to maintain balanced blood sugar to avoid stressing the liver, which is responsible for over five hundred functions in the body. For example, it eliminates excess hormones and filters out toxins. Stable blood sugar is especially critical when you are ridding your body of unwanted bacteria. When the liver is over-burdened, thyroid issues, polycystic ovary syndrome, hormone imbalances, adult acne, high cholesterol, insulin resistance, and more may result. These issues can make it even more difficult to regulate blood sugar levels.

To keep your blood sugar balanced, follow these guidelines:

- Eat three to four small meals a day. Your first meal should be eaten within sixty minutes of waking.
- Each meal or snack should contain a properly sourced protein, healthy carbs (like fruits, veggies, or whole grains), and when possible a healthy fat.
- Never consume a carb by itself since this will spike your blood sugar.

If possible, always consume protein before a carb, caffeine, or refined sugar.

- Enjoy a protein and carb before bed if you find yourself going to sleep hungry. This will help reduce stress on the body throughout the night and also keep blood sugar levels stabilized.
- If you drink alcohol, treat it like a carb. (After all, wine comes from grapes.) It's best enjoyed after a nourishing meal that includes protein, healthy carbs, and healthy fats. This will dramatically reduce any blood sugar spike from the alcohol and help the liver process it.

To unburden the liver and keep its detoxification pathways clear, choose any combination of the following:

Supplement
- berberine
- fulvic acid
- TUDCA (tauroursodeoxycholic acid)

Herbs
- beetroot
- burdock
- dandelion
- milk thistle
- olive leaf
- parsley

Lifestyle habits
- Castor oil packs—Topical castor oil is known to stimulate digestion and promote healthy detoxification of the liver. Placing a pack over your stomach area and letting it rest for thirty to sixty minutes can enhance the detox and promote healthy hormone balance.[2]
- Vibration plate for lymphatic drainage—Standing on the vibrating platform or plate stimulates the muscles to contract about thirty to fifty times a second, which opens up the lymphatic drainage pathway.
- Lymphatic drainage massage—This specific form of massage promotes healthy movement of cells in the lymphatic system, which is a key detoxification system in the body.
- Dry brushing—A body brush with natural bristles can be used on your body to help increase circulation, detox the skin, aid in digestion, and positively stimulate the nervous system.
- Infrared sauna—Spending time in an infrared sauna helps detoxify the liver and promote healthy digestion.
- Morning sun—Spending time outside in the morning helps regulate cortisol, which plays a role in balancing blood sugar.

- Relaxing nighttime routine—Taking time to wind down before bed can help calm the nervous system and promote higher-quality restorative sleep. See page 66 for helpful practices to follow at bedtime.

Once you've tended to these drainage pathways for thirty days, you can continue taking the supplements as you begin the next phase of the protocol.

DAYS 31–60

Eradicate opportunistic bacteria and heal the gut

After working to ensure drainage pathways have been supported and unburdened, you can move into the detox phase, when you'll reduce the bad gut bugs. In addition to eating real foods and practicing other healthy habits, help heal the gut through the following steps:

1. CHOOSE ONE TO TWO ANTIMICROBIALS TO ERADICATE BAD BACTERIA

Antimicrobial supplements
- berberine
- magnesium
- mastic gum

Antimicrobial herbs
- black cumin oil
- black walnut
- goldthread
- Melia

- Mimosa pudica
- Morinda
- wormwood

2. HELP BODY EXPEL BAD BACTERIA AND SOOTHE UPPER GI TRACT

Binder

A binder is a supplement that acts to bind toxins together and help flush them out of the body. It's typically made up of a combination of activated charcoal and bentonite clay, along with fibers and acids like broccoli sprout, apple pectin, and fulvic acid. Binders are an important part of the detoxing process because when you are exposing internal toxic debris by taking antimicrobials, you want the support of a supplement that will essentially go behind the antimicrobials and mop up and move out everything that might be left.

They can be a powerful tool, but it's important not to take these long term. Just as they are effective at removing unwanted bacteria, they can also remove good bacteria, which can disrupt the ecosystem of the microbiome. As a general rule it's beneficial to take a binder during an active detox process, but there likely is no need for a binder afterward. Reach out to your health-care provider for additional support.

To heal and seal the upper GI tract after the detox, choose from the following:

- aloe vera
- colostrum
- deglycyrrhizinated licorice (DGL)
- lemon balm
- L-glutamine

- marshmallow root
- peppermint
- slippery elm

Lifestyle habits
- Engage in physical activity.
- Practice grounding (see page 116).
- Get seven to nine hours of quality sleep per night.
- Continue any practices begun in the previous phase.

Other considerations

Proper hydration

Proper hydration is imperative for optimal health and gut function. Water that has been properly absorbed can move nutrients from cell to cell in the body, eliminate toxic waste, and act as a bone/joint lubricant. Water also increases the brain's ability to process information, so the brain is sensitive to water loss. Constipation, dry mouth, extreme fatigue, frequent headaches, joint pain, and insomnia can be signs of dehydration.[3] In the most extreme instances, it can even lead to brain damage.

How can you ensure you are drinking enough water?

- Drink half your body weight in ounces of water per day.
- For every eight ounces of caffeinated coffee or tea that you consume, I recommend that you drink twelve ounces of water (in addition to your daily quota).
- Ensure your water has electrolytes for maximum absorption. You can do this by adding either flavored electrolyte powder or a pinch of pink sea salt. In either case, it's not necessary to put electrolytes in every glass of water unless you struggle with chronic dehydration

issues. Put enough in your water to make an impact, but not so much that it tastes overly strong. The taste should be pleasurable.

Hormone regulation and sleep

To keep your hormones balanced and working optimally, I recommend the following:

- Manage stress as much as possible.
- Try to match your wake/sleep cycle to the rhythm of the sun as much as possible. Get up early or just before sunrise, and go to bed no later than 9:30 or 10:00 p.m.

DAYS 61–75+

Create a robust host by increasing good gut bugs and replenishing nutrients

- Add in a spore-based probiotic after sixty days (thirty days of drainage, thirty days of eradicating bad bacteria).
- Eat lots of fermented foods like kimchi, kefir, sauerkraut, and kombucha. Please note, however, that if you have a known fungal infection or overgrowth, you'll want to avoid fermented foods as they can contribute to this issue.

DAYS 75+

Transition out while making this a permanent lifestyle change

As you begin making the shift from the Whole-Body Health Protocol into a lasting lifestyle, the following may help:

1. Remember that a whole-foods diet always supports optimal gut health. Stick to these foods as much as possible. While the respective lists are a little tighter for the protocol itself, once you begin the transition phase, you're free to eat any protein, vegetable, fruit, grain, legume, nut, or seed. Just be sure to try to source your food appropriately and wash your produce to remove contaminants. (I combine one cup water with five drops of grapefruit seed extract in a spray bottle and use the mixture to clean fruits and veggies.) Soak your nuts and grains as often as you can.[4]

2. Use the tools in this appendix whenever needed. For instance, if you feel like your drainage pathways are compromised or you become "backed up" while traveling, you may want to use one or more of these tools to help produce movement.

3. Women can use regular support around the time of their monthly cycle. The suggestions in the "Balance Blood Sugar" section on pages 165–166 will be particularly helpful. Chaste tree berry, milk thistle, dandelion, beet, and raspberry leaf can all be effective tools, along with applying a castor oil pack and eating raw carrots.

4. Remember that the goal isn't to live by this protocol for the rest of your life. It's a tool that can be used one to two times per year to maintain a healthy gut garden and regularly defend against unwanted pathogens in a specific way.

5. I recommend that most people continue to take digestive enzymes or bitters at meals. They provide a good defense

against unwanted bacteria and help the body break down foods. Digestive enzymes are generally safe to take on an ongoing basis, but as with other supplements, you should consult with your health-care provider if you are pregnant or nursing, are taking other medications, or have underlying health conditions.

6. When you aren't getting enough sleep or feel more anxious than usual, take a step back and work to be gentle, kind, and tender with yourself. No more slamming it on the treadmill and counting endless calories to see minimal results. You are working with your body for the rest of your life to support it through every stage, season, and stressful life moment.

7. Take these principles and apply them when you travel. Be in control where you can be in control, and let the rest go. If you want to travel and enjoy a once-in-a-lifetime meal, *do it*. You'll never get that opportunity back.

8. If you want further support that is customized to meet your needs, I highly recommend reaching out to a practitioner in your area.

9. You have what it takes; don't overthink it. Your God-given body is beautiful, redeemed, and breathtaking. Cheering for you!

APPENDIX B

Real-Food Recipes

As we explore the beauty of God's goodness through foods He has provided, it's essential to remember that meals are often designed strictly to provide nourishment and proper fuel. Some of my own gut-healthy meals, for instance, consist of two hard-boiled eggs, one piece of fruit, and high-quality protein powder mixed in water, with which I take my supplements.

But other gut-healthy, nourishing meals have a gourmet flair. After all, it's likely that you will have some kind of special event pop up during the seventy-five days of the protocol. You might host or want to provide a special dish for a birthday party, holiday dinner, or bridal shower. It's important to enjoy those moments, but it's also important to be mindful that you are eating foods that will heal and nourish your system during your personal detox. As we've seen, my husband is gifted in the kitchen, and together we have created a few original recipes from whole foods that look and taste great. Each one complies with the guidelines of this protocol and can be thoroughly enjoyed anytime. I hope you enjoy them as much as we do!

FENNEL SALAD

DRESSING
1/4 cup of extra-virgin olive oil
1 1/2 tablespoons lemon juice
2 tablespoons orange juice
3/4 teaspoon minced gingerroot
Salt to taste

SALAD
Few handfuls of salad greens
1/2 fennel bulb, shaved or sliced very thin
1/4 apple, sliced
1/2 cup red onion, sliced
1/4 cup green olives, halved
3 sprigs mint, stems removed
1 teaspoon capers
1 teaspoon fennel leaf from bulb
Zest of 1 lemon
1/4 cup walnuts, crushed

GOAT CHEESE BLEND
1/4 cup soft goat cheese
Zest of 1 orange
1 teaspoon honey

DIRECTIONS

1. Make the dressing: Whisk together olive oil, lemon juice, orange juice, gingerroot, and salt.
2. Assemble salad: Arrange mixed greens on platter. Then layer in fennel bulb, apple slices, red onion, green olives, mint leaves, capers, and fennel leaf.
3. Make goat cheese blend: In a small bowl, stir together goat cheese, orange zest, and honey until well combined.
4. Add clumps of goat cheese blend to salad. Stir salad dressing and drizzle half on salad, reserving the other half.
5. Sprinkle lemon zest and walnuts on salad and serve with remaining dressing if desired.

Makes 4 servings

BEETS TWO WAYS

BEETS
3 yellow beets
3 red beets
Juice of 1 orange
2 teaspoons gingerroot, minced
¼ to ½ cup water
1 teaspoon fresh mint, chopped
2 tablespoons crushed pistachios
Olive oil
Salt

GOAT CHEESE BLEND
¼ cup soft goat cheese
Zest of 1 lemon
1 teaspoon honey

DIRECTIONS
1. Preheat oven to 400 degrees F.
2. Prepare beets by removing stems and washing them. Tear off two pieces of foil, roughly 1 ½ feet each. Place yellow beets on one sheet and red beets on the other. Drizzle with olive oil and add a pinch of salt. Wrap foil around beets, place on sheet pan, and roast 45–60 minutes, or until fork tender.
3. Make goat cheese blend by combining goat cheese, lemon zest, and honey in a small bowl. Stir until well mixed.

4. Remove beets from oven and place in ice bath to cool. Peel cooled beets.
5. Cut red beets into slices. Chill in refrigerator 30–60 minutes before serving.
6. Combine yellow beets, juice from orange, and gingerroot in blender or food processer. Pulse until puree is formed, adding 1/4–1/2 cup of water if necessary to form a puree. Add salt to taste.
7. To assemble, spoon pureed yellow beets on platter, place sliced red beets on top, add chunks of goat cheese blend, and sprinkle all with mint and crushed pistachios.

Makes 4 servings

PROSCIUTTO-WRAPPED DATE APPETIZER

12 dates, pitted
4 slices of prosciutto
12 cashews
1 orange
1/4 cup goat cheese
1 sprig fresh thyme
1 teaspoon honey

DIRECTIONS

1. Preheat oven to 500 degrees F.
2. Stuff and wrap dates: Cut prosciutto into 12 strips. Insert one cashew in each date and wrap with prosciutto.
3. Slice orange in half. Juice one half; peel other half and divide it into orange slices.
4. Place goat cheese into bowl and combine with 1 teaspoon orange juice, thyme leaves, and honey. Mix well.
5. Cover baking sheet with parchment paper. Place dates on baking sheet and roast for 5 minutes.
6. Remove dates from oven and let cool for 5 minutes.
7. Assemble dates by topping them with clumps of goat cheese mixture and one slice of orange.

Makes 4 servings

WATERMELON SALSA AND POACHED SEA BASS

WATERMELON SALSA
2 cups watermelon, cubed
1 cup cantaloupe, cubed
1/2 cucumber, peeled, seeds removed, and chopped
1 red bell pepper, seeds and stem removed, and chopped
1/2 poblano pepper, seeds and stem removed, and chopped
Salt to taste

SEA BASS
4 sea bass fillets, approximately 1 1/2 pounds
1 cup dry white wine
3 sprigs cilantro
Juice of 2 limes

GARNISH
1/4 cup chili roasted pistachios, crushed
1/8 cup cilantro, chopped
Zest of 1 lime
3-inch piece of peeled cucumber, julienned
Salt to taste

DIRECTIONS

1. Preheat oven to 400 degrees F.
2. Combine watermelon, cantaloupe, cucumber, and peppers in food processor or blender. Pulse until well chopped but still chunky. Add salt to taste.
3. Fill a Dutch oven with enough water to cover fish. Add white wine, cilantro, and lime juice. Bring the liquid to a simmer and then put the fish fillets into the water.
4. Place lid on pan and cook 10 minutes, or until fish is flaky and opaque. Fish should pull apart easily with fork.
5. When fish is done, remove from water and place on plate. Top each fillet with approximately 1/4 cup watermelon salsa, a sprinkle of pistachios, cilantro, lime zest, cucumbers, and salt.

Makes 4 servings

ITALIAN SAUSAGE AND PEPPERS WITH CRUSHED TOMATO SAUCE

PEPPERS AND SAUSAGE
6 bell peppers (a mix of red, yellow, and orange), sliced into 1/4-inch strips
1 red onion, sliced into 1/4-inch strips
2 cloves garlic, smashed
1/2 teaspoon fennel seed
1 teaspoon dried oregano
1/4 teaspoon red pepper flakes
Extra-virgin olive oil
Salt and pepper to taste
1 1/2 pounds Italian sausage links

POTATOES
6 Yukon Gold potatoes, quartered
3 cloves garlic, sliced thin
1/4 teaspoon red pepper flakes
1/2 teaspoon oregano
Extra-virgin olive oil
Salt and pepper to taste

SAUCE
1 can crushed tomatoes with juice
3 cloves garlic, minced
1/2 teaspoon dried basil
1 teaspoon red wine vinegar
Salt and pepper to taste

DIRECTIONS

1. Preheat oven to 400 degrees F.
2. On rimmed sheet pan, add peppers, onion, garlic, fennel seed, oregano, red pepper flakes, oil, salt, and pepper. Stir ingredients together and spread them out on the pan. Place sausage on top.
3. On another sheet pan, add ingredients for potatoes. Stir well and spread out on sheet pan.
4. Cook sausage, peppers, and potatoes for 35–45 minutes. The sausage should reach internal temp of 160–170 degrees F. Potatoes should be fork tender.
5. When cooked, remove sausage, peppers, and potatoes and place on plate. Cover and let rest for 5–10 minutes.
6. Prepare sauce by combining tomatoes, garlic, basil, red wine vinegar, and salt and pepper in small saucepan. Bring to simmer on stovetop.
7. Arrange pepper-and-onion mix on platter. Then layer with potatoes, sausage, and sauce.

Makes 4 servings

EASY OVEN-ROASTED OKRA
AND RED PEPPER SHEET PAN

1 pound fresh okra, stems removed; cut into 1/2–3/4
   inch rounds
1/2 red onion, chopped
1 tomato, chopped
1 red bell pepper, seeds and stem removed,
   chopped
1/4 teaspoon coriander
1/4 teaspoon ground green peppercorn
   (or substitute black pepper)
Avocado oil
Salt to taste
Small handful cilantro, chopped

DIRECTIONS
1. Preheat oven to 425 degrees F.
2. Combine okra, onion, tomato, bell pepper,
   coriander, peppercorn, avocado oil, and salt.
   Place parchment paper on rimmed sheet pan,
   followed by the mixture.
3. Roast for 45 minutes. Turn okra over halfway
   through. Okra should be slightly crispy.
4. Remove from oven, garnish with cilantro, and
   serve.

Makes 4 servings

APPENDIX C

Food Lists

We are *not* talking about or thinking about calories during the Whole-Body Health Protocol; instead, we are going to focus on eating nutrient-dense foods that fuel your body properly. Consuming foods that are rich in nutrients will help the body rid itself of toxins and wastes, leading to weight loss that is healthy and sustainable. The following foods, which will optimize the way your body functions, may be included in your diet:

GO-TO FOODS

Protein

It is optimal if these are organic, grass fed, pasture raised, and/or wild caught. If you purchase frozen meats, check the ingredient list to be sure they contain no added sugar.

bacon

bass

beef

bison

bone broth

cheese (raw or low
    pasteurized)

chicken

cod

cured pork

deli meat (organic and properly sourced; void of artificial ingredients and nitrates)

eggs

halibut

kefir

lamb

milk (from cow, goat, or sheep; raw or gently pasteurized) (only if well-tolerated)

salmon

sushi

tuna

turkey sausage

Vegetables

May be enjoyed in unlimited quantities.

alfalfa

amaranth

artichoke

asparagus

avocado

beets

bok choy

broccoli

brussels sprouts

cabbage

carrots

cauliflower

celery

chicory

cucumber

fennel

green onions

greens (e.g., beet greens, collard, dandelion, kale, mustard, turnip)

golden potatoes

herbs (e.g., parsley, basil, cilantro, rosemary, thyme)

jicama

kale

lettuce

mushrooms

okra

olives

onions

parsnips

radishes

rutabaga

sauerkraut (raw)

scallions

snow peas or pea pods

spinach

summer squash

sweet potatoes

Swiss chard	watercress
turnips	zucchini
water chestnuts	

Fruit: limit of one to three servings per day

No fruit is off-limits, but here is a list to get you thinking.

apples	lemons
apricots	limes
bananas	mangoes
blackberries	oranges
blueberries	pineapples
cherries	plantains
coconut	strawberries
grapefruit (small)	watermelon
grapes	

Fats

It's best if these are organic and unrefined.

almonds/almond butter	hazelnuts
avocado	olives
cashews	pecans
coconut butter	pumpkin seeds
coconut flakes	sunflower seeds/
coconut milk	butter
flaxseed	walnuts

Cooking oils

coconut oil/milk/cream	fish/cod liver oil
extra-virgin olive oil	ghee (clarified butter)

Sweetener

raw manuka honey only

Beverages

almond milk (made from nuts and water only)
coconut milk
coffee alternatives (made from mushrooms,
    dandelion root, or chicory)
herbal teas
raw veggie juices (made from the list on pages 188–189)
water (plain or sparkling)

FOODS TO AVOID

All processed foods

Think anything in a box; foods with five or more ingredients; most items on the inside aisles of the grocery store. This includes processed fats like margarine and canola, soybean, corn, safflower, sunflower, cottonseed, and peanut oil.

Beverages

alcohol
caffeine
juice (unless you make your own
    and don't add sweeteners)
protein shakes

Grains and legumes (unless soaked and sprouted appropriately)

Nightshade veggies

If you struggle with inflammation, any kind of autoimmune disease, irritable bowel syndrome, migraines, skin issues, or joint pain, you will want to take this list more seriously.

eggplant
paprika
peppers (green, red, yellow, orange,
   jalapeño, cayenne, pimento)
potatoes (white and red)
tomatoes

Proteins

catfish and other bottom feeders
dairy
peanuts, peanut butter
soy

Sweeteners

Only consume limited amounts of raw manuka honey.

APPENDIX D

Supplements and Healing Foods

You should strive to get most nutrients from food; however, you might also choose to take one or more supplements that target specific aspects of gut health.* Just remember that supplements are just that—intended to fill any gaps. These are additional supplements that can be helpful, but if you'd prefer to stick with whole foods only, that is fine too.

- ashwagandha—improves DHEA (dehydroepiandrosterone) levels, helps with sleep, boosts immunity, and regulates blood sugar; because it targets the stressed gut, often helpful for chronic stress or season of high stress
- collagen peptides—contain essential building blocks to repair damaged intestinal lining; help restore the mucosal lining
- fish oil—provides omega-3 fatty acids, supports adrenal function, and protects against inflammation
- turmeric—reduces inflammation and targets pain/joint issues

---

* Please note: Because every person (and their health history) is different, I recommend that you talk with your doctor before beginning to take supplements. For more information on choosing quality supplements, see pages 160–161.

- vitamin B_{12}—helps restore adrenal function and increase energy
- vitamin C—helps boost immunity and aids in digestion

HEALING FOODS

I highly recommend adding in the following nutrients, as you are able, to support the healing of your gut. There's no need to consume everything from the list every day, however. There is also no formula. If I could choose only one item from this list, I would drink a mug of bone broth daily at any time of the day.

- bone broth—provides rich amounts of collagen (see healing properties of collagen on page 193)
- fermented beverages, such as apple cider vinegar, kvass, and kombucha—help restore good bacteria and aid in digestion
- fermented vegetables, such as sauerkraut, pickled vegetables, and kimchi—provide digestion-enhancing enzymes and good bacteria; help produce stomach acid
- green superfood powder—improves liver function in the detoxification process
- kefir—provides high levels of naturally occurring diverse bacteria
- manuka honey—destroys H. pylori bacteria in the stomach because of its antimicrobial properties
- mushrooms—help balance microbes in the microbiome, boost immune system, detoxify chemicals and heavy metals, and help balance cortisol levels and other stress hormones
- pau d'arco tea—calms the gut
- raw cheese—provides probiotics

APPENDIX E

Guidelines

To help you get started on your healing protocol, I want to suggest what a typical day could look like:

A TYPICAL DAY	
Rise and Reflect	
Timing	Get up early enough that you don't need to rush around. Stress management and meditation will be key during this process. Take ten to sixty minutes to read, write, journal, plan the day ahead, and focus on things you are grateful for. Not only will this help you feel more settled, but your gut will also have time to wake up and start working as it should.
pH	Before you do anything else, prepare a glass of hot lemon water by pouring boiling water into your favorite mug and squeezing in half a lemon. Sip it as you take your vitamin C supplement. The lemon water helps balance the pH levels in your system to get your metabolism going. If you enjoy coffee or hot tea, you can follow the hot lemon water with one of those. (Review the food list for approved types of coffee and tea.)
Food to Go	Pack a nutritious lunch if you will be eating away from home.

A TYPICAL DAY	
Nourish	
Breakfast	Make sure you eat a good breakfast that is filled with protein and healthy fats. This will immediately fuel your system and brain. I generally make a protein smoothie with 1–2 cups of berries, between 1 teaspoon and 1 tablespoon of flax oil, and water. After that, I enjoy a cup of decaf coffee with a splash of coconut milk or homemade almond creamer. This is also when I take my supplements with my first tumbler of water. I drink several tumblers each day, and I add a scoop of electrolytes for added mineral support to one 40-ounce tumbler of water. If you can get out to enjoy the first morning light from the sun, going out for a walk after breakfast will help balance your blood sugar and promote a healthy cortisol rhythm for the day.
Midmorning	Eat a snack. For instance, I often eat two eggs (scrambled, hard-boiled, or fried), breakfast meat, and a mini side salad with 1 cup spinach; eight to ten almonds, cashews, or walnuts; red onion slices; and a drizzle of lemon. After you finish your snack, do something fulfilling, even if just for five minutes. If you have a desk job, look away from your computer, take a lap outside or around your office building, put down your phone, stretch your legs, call a friend, or pray.

A TYPICAL DAY	
Nourish	
Lunch	Fill your lunch with lots of colorful nutrients. Try to include at least one protein, carb, and fat, and eat slowly until you feel full. My lunch normally includes meat like chicken or ground beef and whatever fruits and veggies I have on hand. (I cut up a *ton* of fruits and veggies on Sundays so it's all prepped and ready to pull from the fridge.)
Midafternoon	Repeat midmorning activities if you can. Have a snack, turn away from your computer, etc. I often sip a mug of bone broth and sometimes eat a palm-sized serving of pumpkin seeds and fresh berries.
Dinner	Don't be afraid to try new things, and as long as you're eating from the list of approved foods, don't be concerned about how many calories you're eating. At dinnertime, my family often enjoys grilled fajita meat with grilled veggies or lots of roasted veggies and a cup of rice (when not on a detox) on a bed of greens. We drizzle with homemade sauces and spices to taste.
Evening	If you get hungry after dinner, eat another snack that includes a protein and a carb from the list! When your body tells you it's hungry, it's important to fuel it. I drink an herbal tea designed to help with stress to ease into my bedtime routine.

A TYPICAL DAY	
Healthy Habits	
Chew	Chew your food thoroughly, twenty to thirty times every bite. This cuts down on the amount of work your digestive system has to do and gives your gut a break.
Relax	Try not to eat while standing or driving. Your body needs to be in a relaxed state in order to digest food properly.
Temperature	Try not to eat anything at its coldest temperature. Cold food and drinks force your digestive system to work harder. Not only must it digest, but it also has to regulate your internal temperature. This means no cold produce, water, or leftovers. If you work in an office without a microwave, pull out your lunch ten to thirty minutes before you consume it, and let it reach room temperature before consumption.
Socialize	Spend time with people who bring you life. If any friendships or relationships are not life-giving or are causing tension, pray about them, asking the Lord where you might need to ask for or offer forgiveness or even set boundaries.

A TYPICAL DAY

Healthy Habits

Move	Move your body. Do a workout that you love. If you dread exercise, consider trying something totally new or just go for a ten-minute walk. Don't spend the next forty days beating yourself up about hating to work out or missing a workout. Moving your body is a privilege and should be fun. If it isn't, allow yourself to explore why.
Opt for Outside	Get out in nature. Trees and other plants give off chemicals called phytoncides that will improve your mood and can help if you deal with depression.[1]
Device Breaks	Watch a movie without holding your phone.
Soak	Take a healing bath using things like Epsom salt and lavender oil.
Align	Visit a chiropractor for an alignment to get everything moving properly.

APPENDIX F

FAQs

How can I keep costs down while following this plan?

- Buy meat in bulk and then freeze what you don't use immediately.
- Purchase organic meat and eggs first; then purchase organic produce as your budget allows.
- To cut costs and minimize food waste, shop with a friend and split the grocery bill in half.
- Order curbside pickup from your grocery store if you can. That way you order exactly what you need and won't be tempted to buy impulse items.

What if my family isn't excited about following this plan with me?
When you are passionate about changing your lifestyle to bring about lasting healing, the changes don't happen overnight. It might take time for certain family members to get on board, and that's okay. If they do not want to change their eating habits with you, ask them how they might be willing to support you or compromise. Maybe try cooking separate meals for each other but doing

it together. Maybe clean out a cabinet or a refrigerator shelf just for you that doesn't inconvenience anyone else. It is hard when those you live with are not on the same page, so in such situations I recommend partnering with a friend or a trusted practitioner for additional accountability.

I slipped up for a day (or a week). Should I start over?

I think one meal or even a day that isn't focused on the plan is okay. However, if you needed to veer off the path for a week or longer, I suggest resetting the clock on six weeks, especially if you have sugar cravings, low thyroid, poor sleep quality, or are prone to weight gain. Remember that the body craves consistency, so when you are working to bring healing to the gut, you want to be mindful of anything that might trigger the body negatively. Going back and forth is hard on your hormones, and the gut and hormones are so closely connected that consistency is important to keep blood sugar balanced and to minimize exposure to gut triggers while healing is taking place.

I'm going on vacation in the middle of this. Should I even try to follow this protocol?

Yes! As I've said, there is no perfect time to start. Your interest in this plan was piqued for a reason. Lean into that and do your best. Stick to your own nonnegotiables.

Here are some tips to follow when traveling during the protocol:

- Pack as many sources of travel proteins as you can. Grass-fed protein powders, collagen powder, and beef sticks are my personal favorites.
- Pack as many sources of travel carbs as you can, such as dried fruits and veggies.

- Pack as many sources of travel fats as you can. Dehydrated coconut, nuts, and olives are always go-tos for me.
- When eating out, source the cleanest meat and the best carb (steamed veggies, rice, fruit). If you still feel hungry, choose one of the snack items that you packed.
- Most hotels have refrigerators. If you call ahead, you can usually have one put in your room fairly easily.
- Ration out any supplements that you are taking and put them in a pill box so you can just grab and go.

I like eating salads, but they're cold. Is that okay?
Yes, just pull your salad out of the fridge about ten to fifteen minutes before you eat it.

Should I have dairy?
Stay away from dairy during the protocol. If you can tolerate it, you can reintroduce it during the transition phase.

If yogurt is a protein source that you particularly enjoy, look for coconut or sheep's milk yogurt. We are avoiding cow's milk on this protocol, but sheep's milk yogurt in limited quantities is typically well-tolerated. Try it out and see what works for you! Added ingredients and sugars, even those from real fruit, should be avoided. You can sweeten it with raw manuka honey.

How do I know which brand of supplements to buy?
See pages 160–161 for some ideas, but don't get too hung up on this during the protocol. If you enjoy doing research, look at how the supplement was made, where the ingredients came from, if the ingredients are real or synthetic, and how far the supplement had to travel to get to your grocery store. You will learn more along the way.

Can I have creamer in my coffee?

If your goal is to consume only real foods, you might choose a black coffee alternative and/or decaf and add a small amount of full-fat coconut milk instead. You can also put high-quality protein powder and/or collagen in your coffee for extra metabolism and blood sugar support.

Am I going to feel lousy or get sick when I start this plan?

I can't answer this because I don't know you, but if you've been hooked on sugar and/or caffeine, you may experience withdrawal symptoms. If you are concerned about this, take immune support supplements. Stick with the program and drink lots of water.

Can I follow this plan while nursing/pregnant?

Consult with your physician or health-care provider if you are pregnant or nursing.

What do I do if I'm anxious or scared about starting this plan?

Take some deep breaths, believe in yourself, and be free. Remember, knowledge is power, and it's a privilege to take care of your body. Don't give up when it gets hard; it's not worth losing the improvements you've gained.

Notes

CHAPTER 1: FOOD FOR THOUGHT

1. Joel R. Soza, *Food and God: A Theological Approach to Eating, Diet, and Weight Control* (Eugene, OR: Wipf & Stock, 2009), 7.
2. "The Evolution of Food Production," Brunel, February 17, 2022, https://www.brunel.net/en-au/blog/life-sciences/evolution-of-food-production.
3. Sarah Peters Kernan, "Sugar and Power in the Early Modern World," Newberry Digital Collections for the Classroom, March 18, 2021, https://dcc.newberry.org/?p=16944.
4. "Food Is a Weapon: Nutrition Programs Fight for Victory," Oregon Secretary of State website, accessed October 17, 2023, https://sos.oregon.gov/archives/exhibits/ww2/Pages/services-nutrition.aspx.
5. Anna Diamond, "A Crispy, Salty, American History of Fast Food: Adam Chandler's New Book Explores the Intersection between Fast Food and U.S. History," *Smithsonian*, June 24, 2019, https://www.smithsonianmag.com/history/crispy-salty-american-history-fast-food-180972459/.
6. Martin Wolk, "The Real Cost of Convenience Food," NBC News, January 22, 2003, https://www.nbcnews.com/id/wbna3073326.
7. Malik Altaf Hussain, "Food Contamination: Major Challenges of the Future," *Foods* 5, no. 2 (March 2016): 21, https://doi.org/10.3390/foods5020021.
8. Tom Rawstorne, "Are Your Ready Prepared Fruit & Veg as Healthy as You Think? Tests Show Far Lower Levels of Vitamin C than Unprepared Produce," *Daily Mail*, March 20, 2015, https://www.dailymail.co.uk/news/article-3005061.
9. D. Partridge et al., "Food Additives: Assessing the Impact of Exposure to Permitted Emulsifiers on Bowel and Metabolic Health—Introducing the

FADiets Study," *Nutrition Bulletin* 44, no. 4 (December 2019): 329–349, https://doi.org/10.1111/nbu.12408.

CHAPTER 2: GUT CHECK

1. National Institute of Diabetes and Digestive and Kidney Diseases, "Your Digestive System and How It Works," accessed October 17, 2023, https:// www.niddk.nih.gov/health-information/digestive-diseases/digestive-system -how-it-works.
2. Ifeanyichukwu Ogobuiro et al., "Physiology, Gastrointestinal," *StatPearls* (Treasure Island, FL: StatPearls Publishing, 2023), https://www.ncbi.nlm .nih.gov/books/NBK537103/.

CHAPTER 3: THE NUTS AND BOLTS OF NUTRIENTS

1. Some health-care professionals say that having just one bowel movement every three days is fine, but I disagree. Unless we regularly eliminate the toxins from our environment and food, they will just cycle throughout our system.
2. I first heard this commonly used analogy when I was studying nutrition. See, for example, Anahad O'Connor, "Probiotics, Prebiotics and Postbiotics: The Microbe Garden in Your Gut," *Washington Post*, July 4, 2023, https://www.washingtonpost.com/wellness/2023/07/04 /probiotics-prebiotics-postbiotics-microbiome/.
3. To help stimulate the liver to create more enzymes and bile, consume dandelion root, radishes, and bitter greens. Bile salts are essential for gallbladder function, so if your gallbladder has been removed, consider bile salts to help with digestion.
4. Susan Blum, *The Immune System Recovery Plan: A Doctor's 4-Step Program to Treat Autoimmune Disease* (New York: Scribner, 2013), 182.
5. "Hypochlorhydria," Cleveland Clinic, last reviewed June 27, 2022, https:// my.clevelandclinic.org/health/diseases/23392-hypochlorhydria.
6. I often recommend that clients take a probiotic with at least 50 billion CFUs because their digestive system would benefit from more support. However, because some people cannot tolerate this dose right off the bat, they work up to it by starting with a lower dose.
7. Mershen Govender et al., "A Review of the Advancements in Probiotic Delivery: Conventional vs. Non-Conventional Formulations for Intestinal Flora Supplementation," *AAPS PharmSciTech* 15, no. 1 (February 2014): 29–43, https://doi.org/10.1208/s12249-013-0027-1.
8. Robynne Chutkan, *The Microbiome Solution: A Radical New Way to Heal Your Body from the Inside Out* (New York: Avery, 2015), 174. See also Govender et al., "A Review of the Advancements in Probiotic Delivery."

9. F. Batmanghelidj, *Water for Health, for Healing, for Life: You're Not Sick, You're Thirsty!* (New York: Grand Central Publishing, 2003).

10. Angela Ryan Lee, "What Are Electrolytes?" Verywell Health, January 24, 2022, https://www.verywellhealth.com/electrolytes-5211041; "Electrolytes," Cleveland Clinic, last reviewed September 24, 2021, https://my.clevelandclinic.org/health/diagnostics/21790-electrolytes.

CHAPTER 5: WORK THE (IMMUNE) SYSTEM

1. "10 Germy Surfaces You Touch Every Day," ABC News, September 17, 2008, https://abcnews.go.com/Health/ColdandFluNews/story?id=5727571.

2. Philipp Dettmer, *Immune: A Journey into the Mysterious System That Keeps You Alive* (New York: Random House, 2021), 29.

3. Dettmer, *Immune*, 29.

4. "Antigen," MedlinePlus, reviewed July 19, 2021, https://medlineplus.gov/ency/article/002224.htm.

5. The development of autoimmune disorders is complicated, and genetic predisposition often plays a role. Lifestyle, diet, and environment can influence how genes react, making someone more or less likely to develop an autoimmune disease.

6. Selma P. Wiertsema et al., "The Interplay between the Gut Microbiome and the Immune System in the Context of Infectious Diseases throughout Life and the Role of Nutrition in Optimizing Treatment Strategies," *Nutrients* 13, no. 3 (March 9, 2021): 886, https://doi.org/10.3390/nu13030886.

7. Robynne Chutkan, *The Anti-Viral Gut: Tackling Pathogens from the Inside Out* (New York: Avery, 2022), 76.

8. David Perlmutter, *Brain Maker: The Power of Gut Microbes to Heal and Protect Your Brain—for Life* (New York: Little, Brown and Co., 2015), 104.

9. Edwin McDonald, "What Foods Cause or Reduce Inflammation?" University of Chicago Medicine, September 4, 2020, https://www.uchicagomedicine.org/forefront/gastrointestinal-articles/what-foods-cause-or-reduce-inflammation.

10. "Chronic Stress Can Interfere with Normal Function of the Immune System, Suggests New Research," American Psychological Association press release, November 3, 2002, https://www.apa.org/news/press/releases/2002/11/chronic-stress. See also Gregory E. Miller, Sheldon Cohen, and A. Kim Ritchey, "Chronic Psychological Stress and the Regulation of Pro-Inflammatory Cytokines: A Glucocorticoid-Resistance Model," *Health Psychology* 21, no. 6 (November 1, 2002): 531–541, https://doi.org/10.1037/0278-6133.21.6.531.

11. Jeffrey Rediger, *Cured: Strengthen Your Immune System and Heal Your Life* (New York: Flatiron Books, 2021), 192.
12. Rediger, *Cured*, 193. Italics in the original.
13. Satchin Panda, *The Circadian Code: Lose Weight, Supercharge Your Energy, and Transform Your Health from Morning to Midnight* (New York: Rodale, 2018), 29–30.
14. Eric Suni and Abhinav Singh, "Circadian Rhythm: What It Is, What Shapes It, and Why It's Fundamental to Getting Quality Sleep," Sleep Foundation, updated September 8, 2023, https://www.sleepfoundation .org/circadian-rhythm.
15. Changgui Gu et al., "Network Structure of the Master Clock Is Important for Its Primary Function," *Frontiers in Physiology* 12 (August 16, 2021), https://doi.org/10.3389/fphys.2021.678391.
16. Lana Bandoim, "What Are Hypothalamus Disorders?: Healthy Vs. Abnormal Hypothalamus Functioning," Verywell Health, December 20, 2021, https://www.verywellhealth.com/hypothalamus-disorders-anatomy -function-and-treatment-5201467.
17. Ashna Ramkisoensing and Johanna H. Meijer, "Synchronization of Biological Clock Neurons by Light and Peripheral Feedback Systems Promotes Circadian Rhythms and Health," *Frontiers in Neurology* 6 (June 5, 2015): 128, https://doi.org/10.3389/fneur.2015.00128.
18. National Heart, Lung, and Blood Institute, "How Much Sleep Is Enough?," last updated March 24, 2022, https://www.nhlbi.nih.gov /health/sleep/how-much-sleep.
19. Amy Paturel, "Sleep More, Weigh Less," WebMD, August 14, 2022, https://www.webmd.com/diet/sleep-and-weight-loss.
20. "Serotonin," Cleveland Clinic, last reviewed March 18, 2022, https:// my.clevelandclinic.org/health/articles/22572-serotonin.
21. Natalie G., "How Digestion Affects Your Sleep Quality," Sleep Advisor, updated October 13, 2023, https://www.sleepadvisor.org/sleep-and -digestion/.
22. Markham Heid, "Why Sleep Is So Important for a Healthy Immune System," Everyday Health, March 10, 2023, https://www.everydayhealth .com/sleep/why-sleep-is-so-important-for-a-healthy-immune-system/.
23. John Piper, "Neither Do I Condemn You," March 6, 2011, video, 40:47 (quote begins at 33:18), https://www.desiringgod.org/messages/neither -do-i-condemn-you--3.
24. Piper, "Neither Do I Condemn You" (quote begins at 34:28).

CHAPTER 6: ODD COUPLE

1. Amber J. Tresca, "The Anatomy of the Enteric Nervous System: Regulating Digestion," Verywell Health, updated September 25, 2023, https://www.verywellhealth.com/enteric-nervous-system-5112820.

2. Sherry Lin, "4 Tips to Support the Gut-Brain Connection and Improve Your Gut Health," Foodsmart, July 28, 2021, https://foodsmart.com/blog/the-gut-brain-connection-and-ways-to-support-it.

3. David Perlmutter, *Brain Maker: The Power of Gut Microbes to Heal and Protect Your Brain—for Life* (New York: Little, Brown and Co., 2015).

4. Leon M. T. Dicks, "Gut Bacteria and Neurotransmitters," *Microorganisms* 10, no. 9 (September 14, 2022): 1838, https://doi.org/10.3390/microorganisms10091838.

5. "Amino Acid," Scitable, accessed November 6, 2023, https://www.nature.com/scitable/definition/amino-acid-115/.

6. Jane Sandwood, "The Connection between Protein and Your Mental Health," Mental Health Connecticut, July 9, 2019, https://mhconn.org/nutrition/protein-and-mental-health/.

7. Trudy Scott, *The Anti-anxiety Food Solution: How the Foods You Eat Can Help You Calm Your Anxious Mind, Improve Your Mood, and End Cravings* (Oakland, CA: New Harbinger, 2011), 109.

8. Brian Stanton and Kevin R. Gendreau, "Bioavailability and Nutrient Density: Optimizing Your Diet for More Nutrition," Carb Manager, accessed October 19, 2023, https://www.carbmanager.com/article/y2oy0xaaaminwxtv/bioavailability-and-nutrient-density-optimizing-your.

9. Amy Myers, "The Problem with Grains and Legumes," AmyMyers MD.com, accessed October 19, 2023, https://www.amymyersmd.com/article/problem-grains-legumes.

10. "Gamma-Aminobutyric Acid (GABA)," Cleveland Clinic, last reviewed April 25, 2022, https://my.clevelandclinic.org/health/articles/22857-gamma-aminobutyric-acid-gaba.

11. Research shows that tears release oxytocin and endorphins that can help ease pain. See Leo Newhouse, "Is Crying Good for You?," Harvard Health Publishing, March 1, 2021, https://www.health.harvard.edu/blog/is-crying-good-for-you-2021030122020.

12. Arielle Schwartz, "Connection and Co-Regulation in Psychotherapy," Center for Resilience Informed Therapy, November 6, 2018, https://drarielleschwartz.com/connection-co-regulation-psychotherapy-dr-arielle-schwartz/.

CHAPTER 7: STRESSED OUT

1. Robyne Hanley-Dafoe, "Buckets Full of Stress," *Psychology Today*, July 10, 2023, https://www.psychologytoday.com/us/blog/everyday-resilience/202307/buckets-full-of-stress.

2. American Heart Association, "How Much Sugar Is Too Much?," accessed October 24, 2023, https://www.heart.org/en/healthy-living/healthy-eating/eat-smart/sugar/how-much-sugar-is-too-much; John R. White Jr., "Sugar," *Clinical Diabetes* 36, no. 1 (January 1, 2018): 74–76, https://doi.org/10.2337/cd17-0084.

3. Centers for Disease Control and Prevention, "Get the Facts: Added Sugars," last reviewed November 28, 2021, https://www.cdc.gov/nutrition/data-statistics/added-sugars.html; American Heart Association, "How Much Sugar Is Too Much?"

4. Michael J. Breus, "The Connection between Sugar and Your Gut," *Psychology Today*, December 5, 2019, https://www.psychologytoday.com/us/blog/sleep-newzzz/201912/the-connection-between-sugar-and-your-gut; Michael Lam, Carrie Lam, and Jeremy Lam, "Low Stomach Acid: How to Heal the Issue You Didn't Know You Had," Dr. Lam Coaching, accessed October 20, 2023, https://www.drlamcoaching.com/blog/low-stomach-acid/.

5. Casey Seidenberg, "Why We Crave Sugar, and How to Beat the Habit," *Washington Post*, January 30, 2018, https://www.washingtonpost.com/lifestyle/wellness/explaining-the-siren-song-of-sugar-and-how-to-beat-the-habit/2018/01/26/8a9557f8-f7ae-11e7-a9e3-ab18ce41436a_story.html.

6. Jill Neimark, "A Protein in the Gut May Explain Why Some Can't Stomach Gluten," NPR, December 9, 2015, https://www.npr.org/sections/thesalt/2015/12/09/459061317/a-protein-in-the-gut-may-explain-why-some-cant-stomach-gluten.

7. Enzo Spisni et al., "Differential Physiological Responses Elicited by Ancient and Heritage Wheat Cultivars Compared to Modern Ones," *Nutrients* 11, no. 12 (November 26, 2019): 2879, https://doi.org/10.3390/nu11122879.

8. F. Batmanghelidj, *Water for Health, for Healing, for Life: You're Not Sick, You're Thirsty!* (New York: Grand Central Publishing, 2003), 57–60.

9. World Health Organization, "Stress," February 21, 2023, https://www.who.int/news-room/questions-and-answers/item/stress.

10. Anna Cláudia Calvielli Castelo Branco et al., "Role of Histamine in Modulating the Immune Response and Inflammation," *Mediators of Inflammation* (August 27, 2018): article ID 9524075, https://doi.org/10.1155/2018/9524075.

11. Nedra Glover Tawwab, *Set Boundaries, Find Peace: A Guide to Reclaiming Yourself* (New York: TarcherPerigee, 2021), 5.

12. Henry Cloud and John Townsend, *Boundaries: When to Say Yes, How to Say No to Take Control of Your Life* (Grand Rapids, MI: Zondervan, 1992), 53.
13. Tawwab, *Set Boundaries, Find Peace*, 103–104.
14. Logan Hailey, "How to Set Boundaries: 5 Ways to Draw the Line Politely," Science of People, accessed October 20, 2023, https://www.scienceof people.com/how-to-set-boundaries/.

CHAPTER 8: THE MISSING LINK

1. Beth Shaw, "When Trauma Gets Stuck in the Body," *Psychology Today*, October 23, 2019, https://www.psychologytoday.com/us/blog/in-the -body/201910/when-trauma-gets-stuck-in-the-body.
2. Saul McLeod, "John Bowlby's Attachment Theory," Simply Psychology, July 5, 2023, https://www.simplypsychology.org/bowlby.html.
3. Robert S. Feldman, *Development across the Life Span* (Upper Saddle River, NJ: Pearson Education, 2020), 189–190.
4. Courtney E. Ackerman, "What Is Attachment Theory? Bowlby's 4 Stages Explained," PositivePsychology.com, April 27, 2018, https://positive psychology.com/attachment-theory/; see also Kendra Cherry, "What Is Attachment Theory? The Importance of Early Emotional Bonds," Verywell Mind, updated February 22, 2023, https://www.verywellmind.com/what -is-attachment-theory-2795337.
5. The statements with arrows from Curt Thompson, *Anatomy of the Soul: Surprising Connections between Neuroscience and Spiritual Practices That Can Transform Your Life and Relationships* (Carol Stream, IL: Tyndale Refresh, 2010), 116.
6. The description of each adult from Morgan Mandriota, "Here Is How to Identify Your Attachment Style," PsychCentral, October 13, 2021, https:// psychcentral.com/health/4-attachment-styles-in-relationships#disorganized -attachment.
7. "Cortisol," Cleveland Clinic, last reviewed December 10, 2021, https:// my.clevelandclinic.org/health/articles/22187-cortisol.
8. Robert K. Ross, "When Time Doesn't Heal All Wounds," TEDx Talk, filmed at Ironwood State Prison, June 1, 2014, video, 13:07 (quote starts at 3:13), https://www.youtube.com/watch?v=dsCNuB_KBUw.
9. Ross, "When Time Doesn't Heal All Wounds," (quote starts at 6:04).
10. Wendy Menigoz et al., "Integrative and Lifestyle Medicine Strategies Should Include Earthing (Grounding): Review of Research Evidence and Clinical Observations," *Explore* 16, no. 3 (May–June 2020): 152–160, https://doi.org/10.1016/j.explore.2019.10.005.
11. For more on this, see Peter A. Levine, *Waking the Tiger: Healing Trauma* (Berkeley, CA: North Atlantic Books, 1997); Bessel van der Kolk, *The Body Keeps the Score: Brain, Mind, and Body in the Healing of Trauma*

(New York: Penguin, 2014); and Hillary L. McBride, *The Wisdom of Your Body: Finding Healing, Wholeness, and Connection through Embodied Living* (Grand Rapids, MI: Brazos Press, 2021).

CHAPTER 9: SLOW DOWN

1. "Enzymes," Cleveland Clinic, last reviewed May 12, 2021, https://my .clevelandclinic.org/health/articles/21532-enzymes; Morgan Denhard, "Digestive Enzymes and Digestive Enzyme Supplements," Johns Hopkins Medicine, accessed October 23, 2023, https://www.hopkinsmedicine.org /health/wellness-and-prevention/digestive-enzymes-and-digestive-enzyme -supplements.
2. Ololade Akinfemiwa, Muhammad Zubair, and Thiruvengadam Muniraj, "Amylase," National Library of Medicine, updated November 10, 2022, https://www.ncbi.nlm.nih.gov/books/NBK557738/.
3. Denhard, "Digestive Enzymes and Digestive Enzyme Supplements."
4. Nor Amira Syahira Mohd Azmi et al., "Cortisol on Circadian Rhythm and Its Effect on Cardiovascular System," *International Journal of Environmental Research and Public Health* 18, no. 2 (January 14, 2021): 676, https://doi.org/10.3390/ijerph18020676.
5. John Mark Comer, *The Ruthless Elimination of Hurry: How to Stay Emotionally Healthy and Spiritually Alive in the Chaos of the Modern World* (Colorado Springs: WaterBrook, 2019), 148, 155. Italics in the original.
6. Comer, *The Ruthless Elimination of Hurry*, 149. Italics in the original.
7. Nida Tabassum Khan, "Coriander Seeds in Diet," *Journal of Advances in Plant Biology* 1, no. 2 (January 9, 2019): 13–16, https://doi.org/10.14302 /issn.2638-4469.japb-18-2565.
8. Elizabeth Klein, "The Manna and Coriander Seed," *Faith & Culture*, June 15, 2020, https://www.faithandculture.com/home/2020/6/15/the-manna -and-coriander-seed.

CHAPTER 10: FEAST OF HIS FAITHFULNESS

1. John Piper, "Ingredients for a Theology of Feasting," *Ask Pastor John* episode 1687, October 4, 2021, https://www.desiringgod.org/interviews /ingredients-for-a-theology-of-feasting.
2. Joy L. Arroyo, "John Wesley's Empowered Regimen: Cultivating Health and Sanctification," *Wesley and Methodist Studies* 13, no. 2 (May 1, 2021): 154–174, https://doi.org/10.5325/weslmethstud.13.2.0154.
3. Jay Wilson, "What Happens to Your Body When You Eat the Same Thing Every Day," Health Digest, updated April 10, 2022, https://www.health digest.com/670007/.

APPENDIX A: WHOLE-BODY HEALTH PROTOCOL

1. David C. Strubler, "Breaking and Making Habits," *Psychology Today*, January 1, 2020, https://www.psychologytoday.com/us/blog/doesnt-get-any-better/202001/breaking-and-making-habits.
2. Noreen Iftikhar, "How to Make and Use Castor Oil Packs," Healthline, December 17, 2019, https://www.healthline.com/health/castor-oil-pack.
3. F. Batmanghelidj, *Water: For Health, for Healing, for Life: You're Not Sick, You're Thirsty!* (New York: Grand Central Publishing, 2003), 60.
4. Meredyth Fletcher, "Could Soaking Nuts, Seeds, Grains or Beans Improve My Digestion?," Karpós Wellness, August 7, 2021, https://www.karposwellness.com/gut/could-soaking-my-nuts-seeds-improve-digestion/.

APPENDIX E: GUIDELINES

1. Jane Marsh, "4 Phytoncides Benefits: How Trees Improve Our Health," environment.co, February 24, 2023, https://environment.co/phytoncides-benefits/.

About the Author

MEREDYTH FLETCHER is a nutritional therapy practitioner with master's degrees in clinical mental health counseling as well as theological and biblical foundations. She is the founder and owner of Karpós Wellness, where she combines her extensive knowledge of the body and mind to help clients of all ages with health issues, trauma, anxiety, depression, and eating disorders to find the root causes that may be driving their unwanted mental and physical symptoms. She believes that God created our bodies to know how to heal themselves, and she studies the brain and the gut to work with clients holistically from a biblical foundational perspective to achieve healing from the inside out. Visit her at karposwellness .com for more resources.

Meredyth and her husband, Daniel, live in Texas. They enjoy cooking, entertaining, and hanging out with their two young sons.

Tyndale | REFRESH

Think Well. Live Well. Be Well.

Experience the flourishing of your mind, body, and soul with Tyndale Refresh.

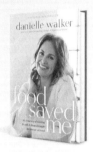
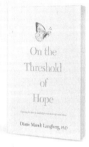
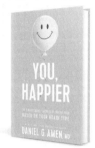
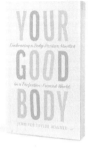

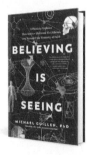
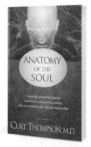
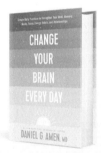
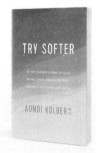

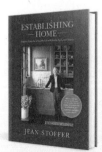
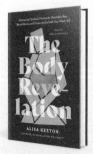
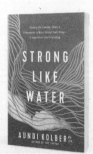
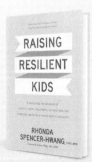